Liver Cirrhosis - Debates and Current Challenges

Edited by Georgios Tsoulfas

Published in London, United Kingdom

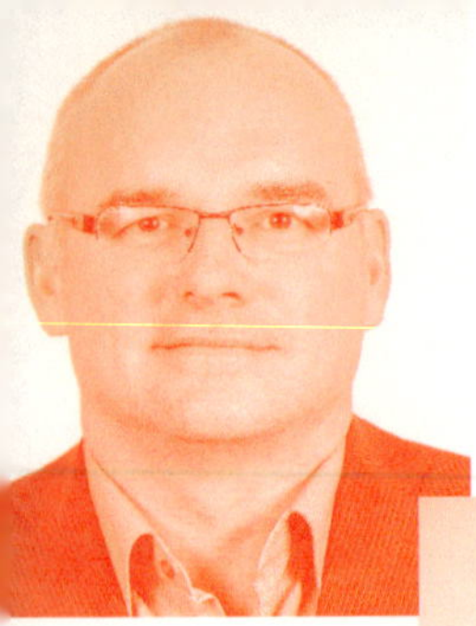
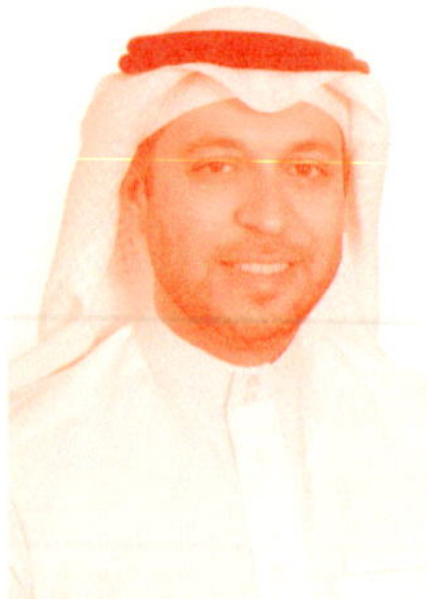
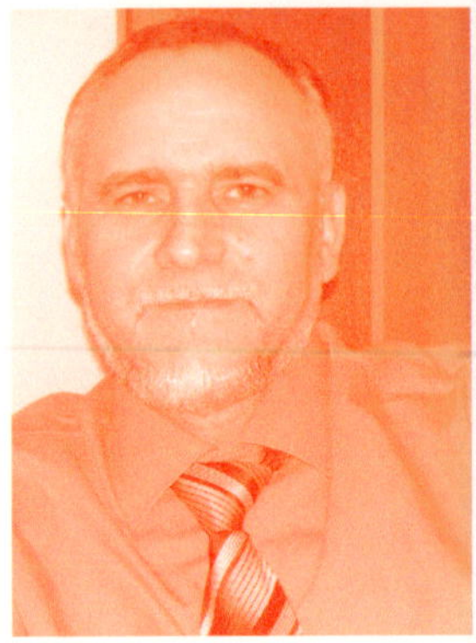
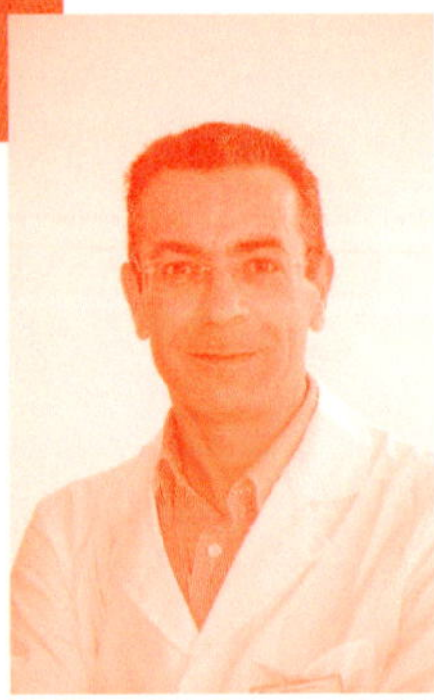
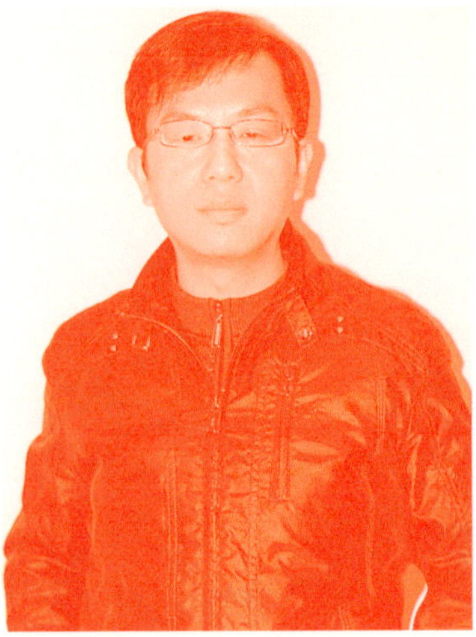
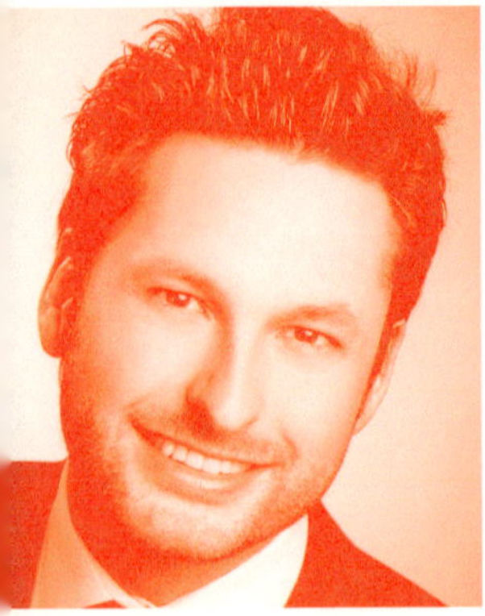
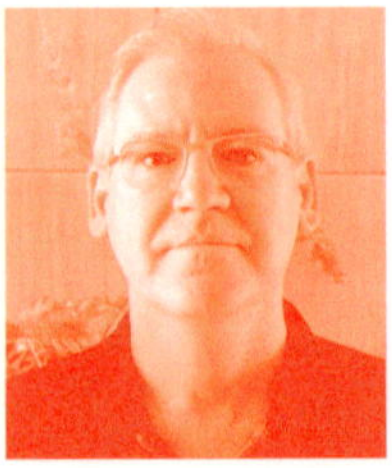

IntechOpen

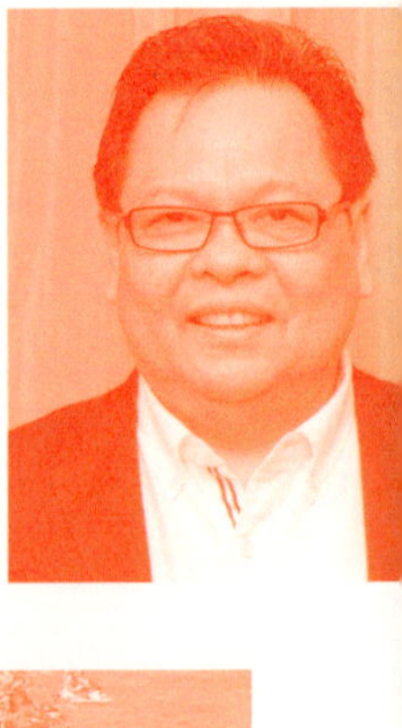
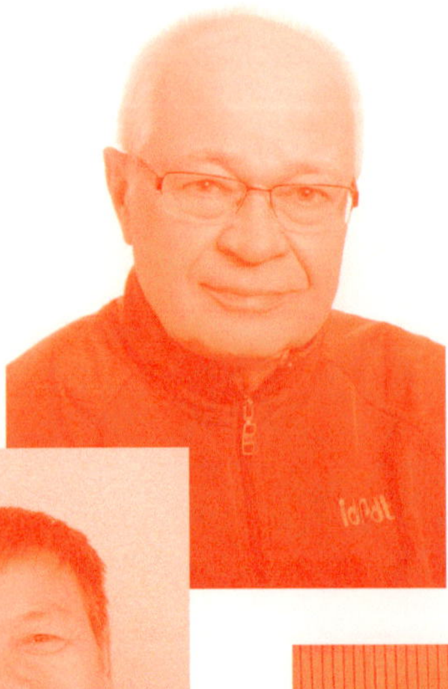
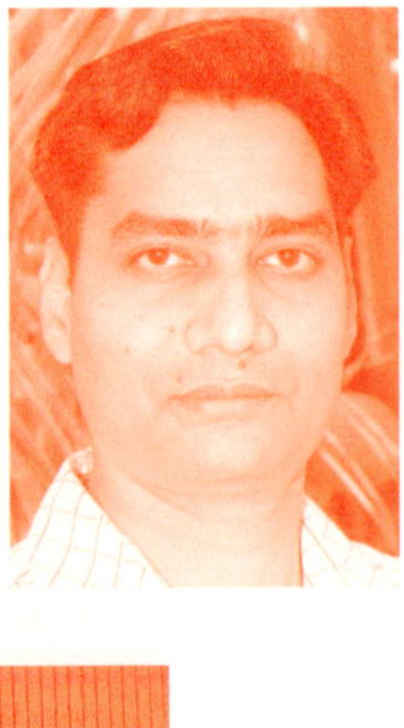
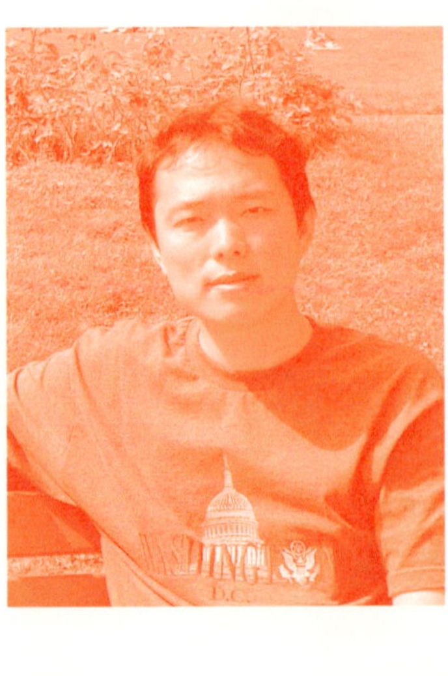
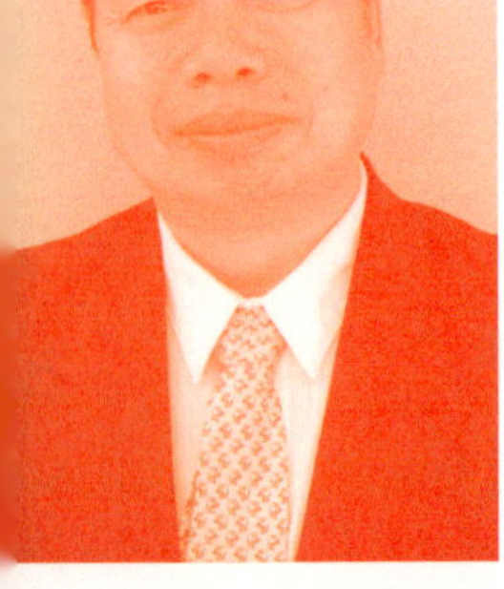
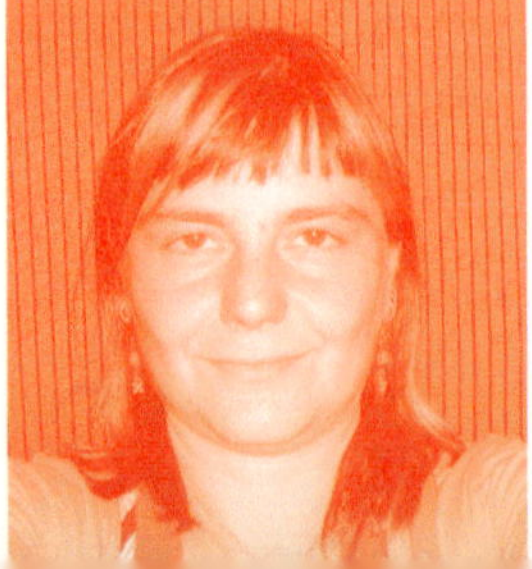

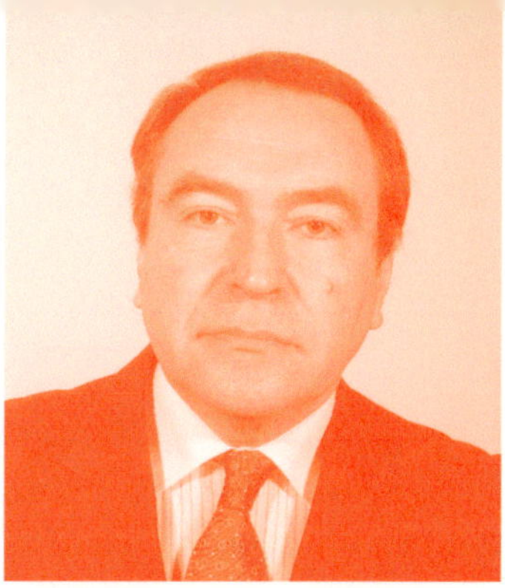
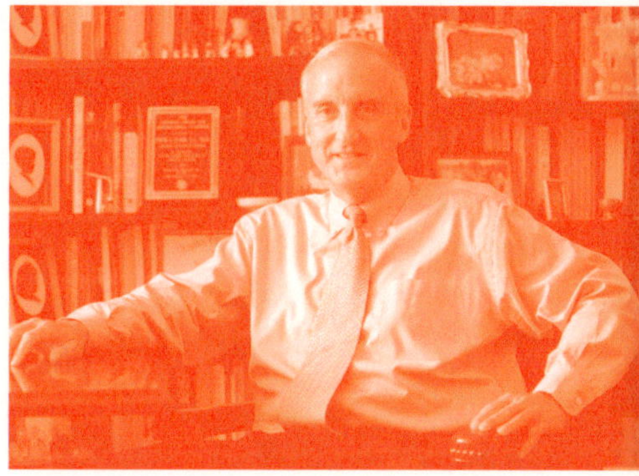
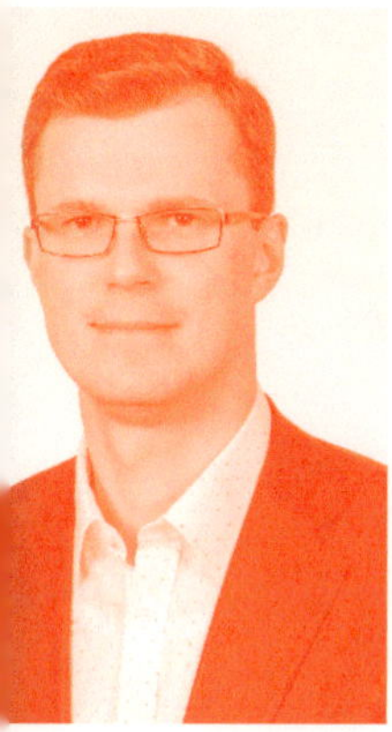
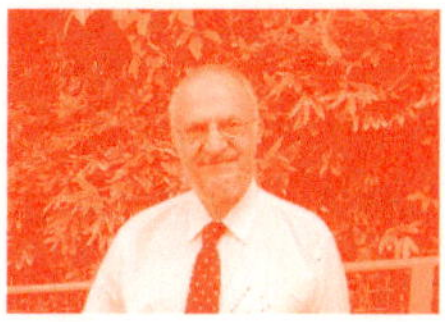
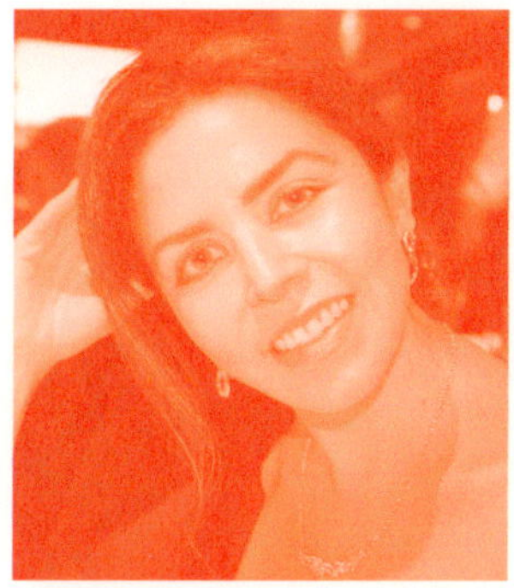

Supporting open minds since 2005

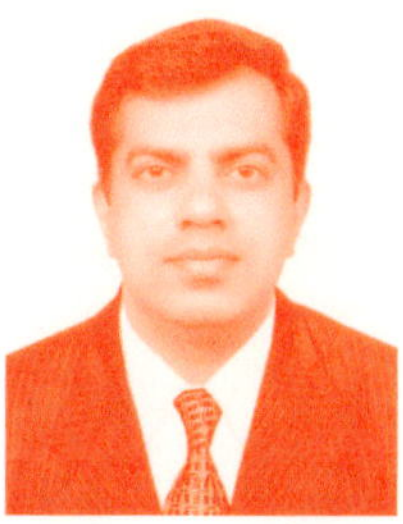
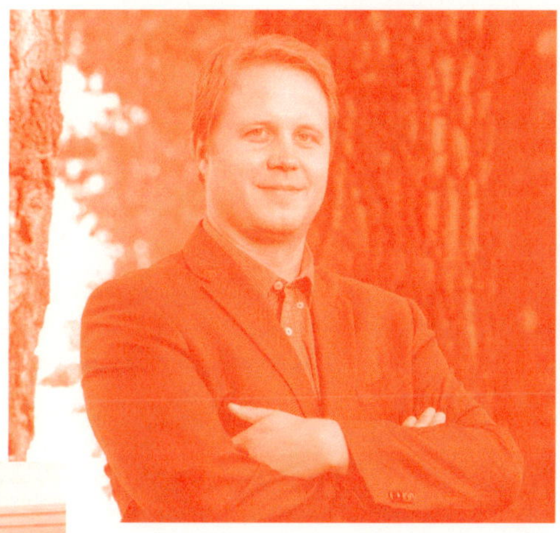
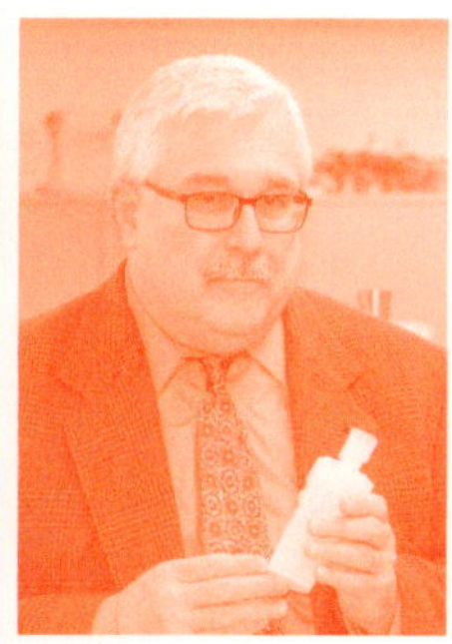
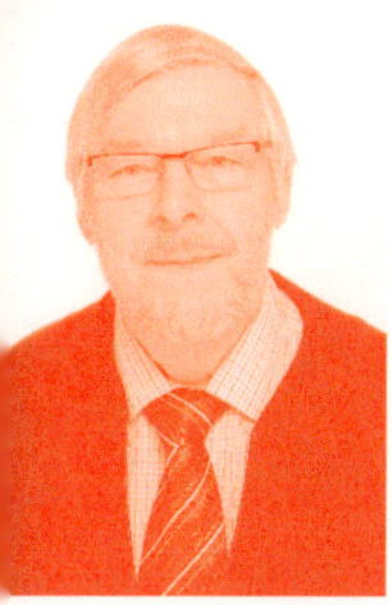
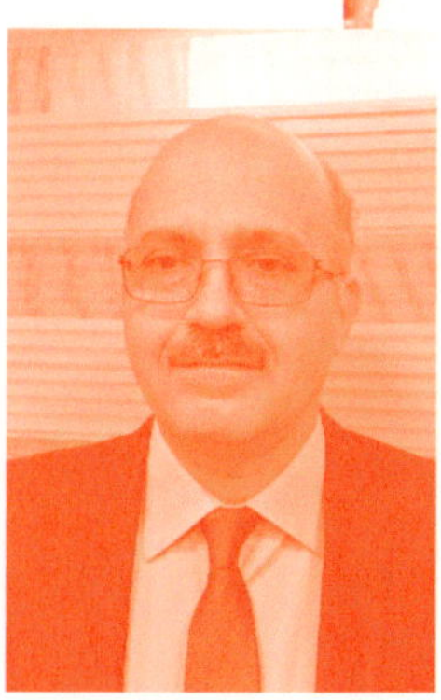
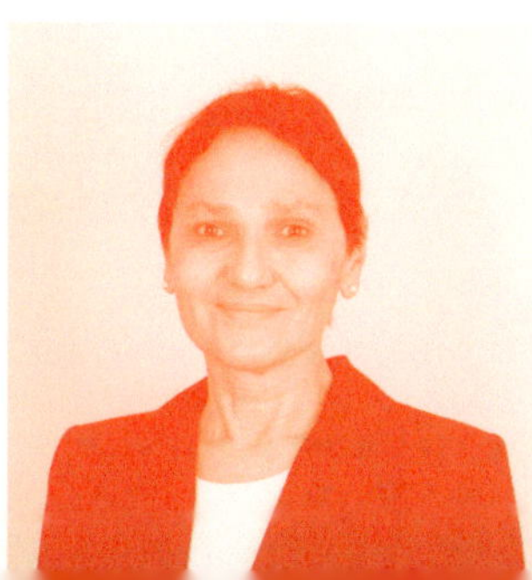
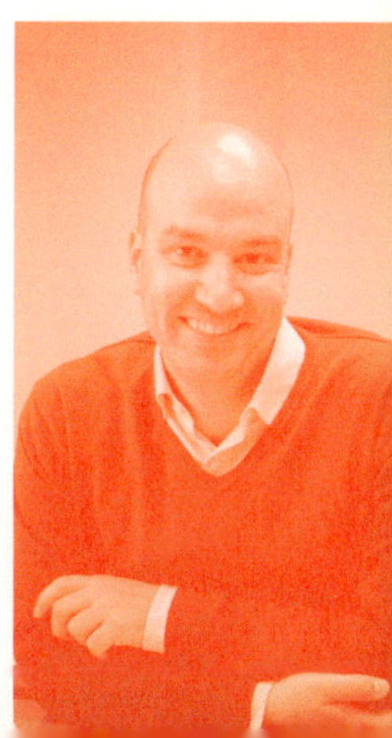

Liver Cirrhosis - Debates and Current Challenges
http://dx.doi.org/10.5772/intechopen.81279
Edited by Georgios Tsoulfas

Contributors
Alexander Vitin, Leonard Azamfirei, Dana Tomescu, Victoria Chagoya De Sanchez, Félix Recillas-Targa, Mariana Domínguez-López, Gabriela Velasco-Loyden, Rebeca Pérez-Cabeza De Vaca, Nuria Guerrero-Celis, Jesús Rafael Rodríguez-Aguilera, Lejla Čalkić, Marco Antonio Lopez Hernandez, Consolato Maria Sergi, Gabriela Gutierrez-Reyes, Moises Martinez-Castillo, David Kershenobich, Linda Muñoz Espinosa, José Luis Pérez Hernández, Paula Cordero Perez, Carolina Guzman, Jacqueline Cordova-Gallardo, Francisco Sanchez-Avila, Eduardo Montalvo-Jave, Daniel Santana-Vargas, Fatima Higuera-De La Tijera, Luis Very-Pineda, Dorothy Rosique-Oramas, Boris Fishman, Vladimir Kulikov, Mikhail Yukhno, Spartak Turmakhanov, Carmen Peralta, Maria Eugenia Cornide Petronio, Mariana Mendes-Braz, Mónica B. Jiménez-Castro, Jordi Gracia-Sancho, Aziza Ajlan, Shatha Al-Muhaideb

First published in London, United Kingdom, 2019 by IntechOpen
IntechOpen is the global imprint of INTECHOPEN LIMITED, registered in England and Wales, registration number: 11086078, The Shard, 25th floor, 32 London Bridge Street
London, SE19SG - United Kingdom
Printed in Croatia

British Library Cataloguing-in-Publication Data
A catalogue record for this book is available from the British Library

Additional hard copies can be obtained from orders@intechopen.com

Liver Cirrhosis - Debates and Current Challenges
Edited by Georgios Tsoulfas
p. cm.
Print ISBN 978-1-78923-885-3
Online ISBN 978-1-78923-886-0
eBook (PDF) ISBN 978-1-83880-445-9

For EU product safety concerns:
IN TECH d.o.o., Prolaz Marije Krucifikse Kozulić 3, 51000 Rijeka, Croatia, info@intechopen.com or visit our website at intechopen.com.

Meet the editor

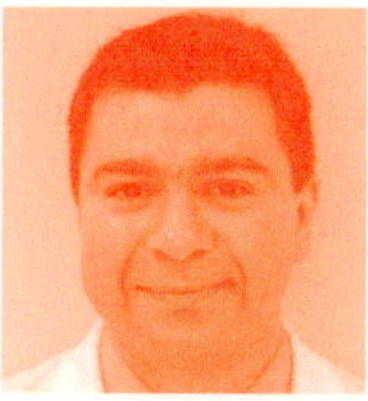

Dr. Georgios Tsoulfas received his medical degree from Brown University School of Medicine and completed his general surgery residency at the University of Iowa Hospitals and Clinics, as well as a transplant research fellowship at the Starzl Transplant Institute at the University of Pittsburgh. He then completed a two-year transplantation surgery fellowship at the Massachusetts General Hospital, Harvard Medical School, and then joined the Division of Solid Organ Transplantation and Hepatobiliary Surgery at the University of Rochester Medical Center as an assistant professor of surgery. He has currently moved back to Greece, where he is an associate professor of surgery at the Aristotle University of Thessaloniki. He has published more than 90 papers in peer-reviewed journals and in PubMed, as well as 29 book chapters. He is a reviewer for more than 40 international journals and is on the editorial boards of several others.
He is currently the Vice Chair of the International Relations Committee of the American College of Surgeons and the World President of the International College of Surgeons.

Contents

Preface

Liver cirrhosis represents the ultimate state of hepatic dysfunction, where a variety of different etiologies lead to the same state of liver failure. The complex nature of the various etiologies, as well as the critical role of hepatic physiology, necessitate a multimodal approach towards diagnosis and management, especially since it is a disease affecting millions of patients of all ages around the globe. It is understandable that during this process, several debates arise, which ultimately have led to significant contributions in the management of liver cirrhosis.

This book provides an overview of all the above with chapters presenting the different etiologies of cirrhosis, the significant complications seen in these patients requiring complex management, as well as the issue of liver transplantation, which remains the ultimate cure. Its value lies in the fact that the authors present us with their distilled wisdom, which is the result of substantial experience and daily involvement in this most difficult field of medicine and surgery.

Overall, this book should be a useful resource for any physician, whether they are in training or in practice, treating patients with hepatic diseases.

Georgios Tsoulfas, MD, PhD, FICS, FACS
Associate Professor of Surgery,
Aristotle University of Thessaloniki,
Thessaloniki, Greece

Section 1

Etiology of Cirrhosis

Chapter 1

Noninvasive Biomarkers for the Diagnosis of Liver Fibrosis and Cirrhosis

Dorothy Rosique-Oramas, Moises Martinez-Castillo, Carolina Guzman, José Luis Pérez Hernández, Jacqueline Cordova-Gallardo, Luis Very-Pineda, Fatima Higuera-De La Tijera, Daniel Santana-Vargas, Eduardo Montalvo-Jave, Francisco Sanchez-Avila, Paula Cordero Perez, Linda Muñoz-Espinosa, David Kershenobich and Gabriela Gutiérrez-Reyes

Abstract

The clinical importance of monitoring liver fibrosis lies in the morbidity and mortality of the chronic liver diseases in relation to the stage and progression of fibrosis. Whether the fibrosis stabilizes or regresses depends on the specific treatment. Liver biopsy, the current standard for the diagnosis, has implicit limitations due to sampling heterogeneity. There are noninvasive imaging methods, such as transient elastography that measures the stiffness of the liver, but it has some limitations (feasibility and unreliability), particularly in obese patients. FibroTest is the most widely used noninvasive serological method worldwide which is efficacious in the extreme stages of fibrosis, but these methods cannot discern intermediate stages. Liver fibrosis is a dynamic response that involves multiple cellular and molecular events with an excessive deposit of extracellular matrix. Even though there is much information on the pathophysiology of fibrosis, that knowledge is still incomplete, greatly hindering the development of both an accurate treatment and a noninvasive diagnostic method with adequate sensitivity for all the stages of fibrosis. It is known that IGFBP participates in liver homeostasis, and thus these proteins can be used as serum biomarkers during the progression of liver fibrosis in chronic hepatitis C.

Keywords: liver fibrosis, inflammation, fibrolysis, noninvasive diagnosis

1. Introduction

The etiologic factors that mainly induce liver fibrosis are alcoholic liver disease (ALD), chronic hepatitis C (CHC), and nonalcoholic fatty liver disease (NAFLD). Fibrogenic response can be organized in four different phases according to damage evolution: activation, production of extracellular matrix proteins (ECM), and deposition and degradation of ECM by hepatic stellate cells (HSCs) [1]. The inefficient resorption and control of ECM components promote the establishment and progression of fibrosis inducing the distortion in the architecture of the hepatic parenchyma.

Moreover, the regulation of wounding response is orchestrated by complex activities within different cells that include HSC, macrophages, myofibroblasts, cells derived from bone marrow, and fibrocytes [1–3]. The main type of ECM proteins produced by HSC comprises collagens, fibronectin, laminin, hyaluronan, proteoglycan, and other elements [3, 4]. It has been extensively reported that liver fibrosis progresses to cirrhosis in 20% of patients; furthermore, if the damage is not controlled, approximately 10% of people can progress to carcinoma hepatocellular, which usually causes death in all the cases [5].

The clinical importance of monitoring liver fibrosis progression is correlated with the reduction of morbidity and mortality of the chronic liver diseases [6]. Whether the fibrosis stabilizes or regresses depends on the specific treatment of the underlying disease, and the grade of fibrosis is a treatment indicator [4]. The clinical evidence documenting the fate of HSC during fibrosis regression in humans is limited, compared to the extensive evidence in animal models [4, 6, 7]. Promising studies showed strong evidence that the opportune and precise identification of the etiology and degree of liver fibrosis could be crucial for decision-making in the management and treatment.

Liver biopsy has been considered the keystone for the diagnosis of fibrosis and inflammation, necrosis, and iron deposition [8]; however, this invasive procedure has implicit important limitations due to sampling heterogeneity and possible surgical complications, variability in the interpretation by pathologists, elevated costs, and the difficulty of tracking the evolution of the disease [9, 10]. Furthermore, biopsy is not recommended in patients with ascites, coagulopathy, diabetes, metabolic syndrome, and ALD [11–13]. For these reasons, in the last years, the medical and research groups have evaluated novel noninvasive strategies to discriminate the liver pathologies.

2. Diagnosis of liver fibrosis

Noninvasive measures of liver fibrosis have streamlined the management of patients with CHC [6]. Imageology methods, such as transient elastography (FibroScan™), which measures the stiffness of the liver, have received great acceptance by clinicians and patients. Clinical trials showed that FibroScan results, which are expressed in kPa, reported similar results to that of METAVIR score during biopsy interpretation of liver fibrosis in patients with CHC [10]. Moreover, this procedure has also been validated in chronic hepatitis B, NAFLD, alcoholic liver disease, primary biliary cirrhosis, and primary sclerosing cholangitis [14, 15]. However, this methodology also has some limitations such as feasibility and unreliability, particularly in obese patients or under the circumstances of limited operator experience [16]. Furthermore, it is important to consider that this strategy is contraindicated during pregnancy, ascites, and implanted cardiac pacemaker patients [10].

A variety of "direct" serum markers reflecting ECM turnover (fibrogenesis and fibrolysis) and/or fibrogenic cell changes have been developed and used clinically [17]. In this sense, the multiple analyses of proteins and clinical trials provide valuable information of liver stage. FibroTest index is within the most accepted worldwide noninvasive serological method in the diagnosis of liver fibrosis by CHC, CHB, and NAFLD [17]. For this analysis are computed five surrogate parameters:

total bilirubin, haptoglobin, gamma-glutamyltranspeptidase (GGT), alpha2-macroglobulin, and apolipoprotein-A. It is important to mention that the validation of any surrogate parameter needs to be validated by the calculation of the area under the receiver operating characteristic curve (AUROC) using liver biopsy as reference [8]. Systematic analysis of several studies revealed that FibroTest displayed an excellent discrimination to identify cirrhosis with AUROC = 0.90 but showed a lesser ability to identify ≥F2 fibrosis stages (AUROC = 0.81). The authors conclude that this index is not ready to substitute liver biopsy in the intermediate stages [18]. Additionally, some limitations such as cost and external validation are documented.

Even though there is much information on the pathophysiology of fibrosis, that knowledge is still incomplete, greatly hindering the development of both an accurate treatment and a noninvasive diagnostic method with adequate sensitivity for all the stages of fibrosis. Such a method must also be able to be performed with the necessary frequency to establish disease progression or regression, as well as the changes that occur in the processes, such as chronic inflammation, fibrogenesis, and fibrolysis. Based on our knowledge of fibrosis pathogenesis, attention is now directed towards strategies for antifibrotic therapies and regulatory challenges for conducting clinical trials with these agents. New therapies are attempting to: (1) control or cure the primary disease or reduce tissue injury; (2) target receptor-ligand interactions and intracellular signaling; (3) inhibit fibrogenesis; and (4) promote resolution of fibrosis. Progress is urgently needed in validating noninvasive markers of fibrosis progression and regression that can supplant biopsy and shorten the duration of clinical trials. Both scientific and clinical challenges remain, however, in the past three decades of steady progress in knowledge liver fibrosis.

This entails analyzing the molecules involved in these processes along with the participation of proteins such as insulin-like growth factor binding proteins (IGFBPs). Recently, IGFBP-1 and insulin-like growth factor (IGF) have been proposed as markers for advanced fibrosis in NAFLD [19]. However, the completed evaluation of IGFBPs in liver diseases is not fully understood.

3. Insulin-like growth factor (IGF) complex

The IGF is a family of proteins with high sequence homology to insulin. The IGF system functions as an endocrine, paracrine, and autocrine regulatory axis for cell proliferation, survival, and apoptosis in different types of cells [20]. In general, the IGF system consists of two surface receptors (IGF1R and IGF2R), two ligands (IGF-1 and IGF-2), and a family of IGFBPs [20, 21].

Liver is the main source of IGFs but its highest concentrations are found in the blood. Both IGF-1 and -2 forms can be detected in small amounts in the kidney and other tissues of different species, for example, in the rat, IGF-I has been detected in serum, milk, amniotic fluid, and bile; it has also been detected in human adult bile [22]. In some experiments, it has been found that IGF-1concentrations are higher in bile of neonatal rats than in the adult rats. Thus, it is believed that IGF-I in bile should have an important role in the development of gastrointestinal tract. However, the precise role and the presence or absence of IGFs and IGFBPs in bile have not yet been clearly defined. The biosynthesis of IGFs depends mainly on the levels of growth hormone (GH), insulin, prolactin, and an adequate nutrition stimulus. In contrast, estrogens and cortisol can antagonize their formation [23].

The production of IGF-1 is stimulated by GH, which is secreted by somatotropic cells in the adenohypophysis. The hepatocytes present GH receptors that are stimulated by this hormone and in a consequence an increase in the transcription of the IGF-1 gene is triggered. IGF-1 inhibits GH secretion either directly acting on the pituitary or indirectly by stimulating the hypothalamic secretion of somatostatin which, in turn, inhibits the release of GH. In this way, a negative feedback loop GH-IGF-1 is established [21, 23].

IGFBPs play important roles in the bioavailability of circulating IGF-I, and their synthesis is under metabolic and hormonal control. Their functions can be summarized as follows: (1) they act as protein carriers in serum and control the influx of IGF-I from the vascular space to the tissues. (2) They prolong the half-life of IGF-I and regulate its metabolism. (3) They provide temporal localization of IGF-1 with the aim to be available under specific requirements. (4) They modulate the interaction of IGF-I with its receptor, thus acting as indirect control of the biological actions of IGF-I.

At present, different types of IGFBPs have been described that are mainly produced by hepatocytes and secreted into the blood serum. They can be a high affinity for binding IGFs (IGFBP-1 to IGFBP-6) or a low affinity (IGFBP-7 among others). Normal serum IGF-I levels are approximately 40 nmol/L, and 99% of circulating IGF-Iis was estimated to be associated with the different IGFBPs, mainly IGFBP-3 [23–25].

In recent years, these proteins have gained great attention due the association as biomarkers in different pathologies [25].

4. IGFBPs and liver fibrosis

An increase in IGFBP-1 levels has been observed during nonalcoholic liver disease and cirrhosis of the liver. At the same time, serum IGFBP-3 concentrations are low, correlating with the severity of liver dysfunction, and signifying poor prognosis in hepatocellular carcinoma (HCC) [26]. In *in vitro* studies, IGFBP-7 expression has been found to hepatocyte apoptosis and HSC activation [27, 28]. In relation to the participation of IGFBP-2, -5 and -6, there is little evidence of their concentrations in serum and the possible association with liver diseases. Nevertheless, those proteins can inhibit angiogenesis (IGFBP-4) [29], regulate the role of TNF-α, tumor growth, and an increased expression in pulmonary and liver fibrosis (IGFBP-5) [30, 31] and promote prostate cancer cell migration (IGFBP-6) [22, 32]. The available information about the role, tissue production, and dependent and independent functions of IGFBPS as well as their regulation in related liver pathologies is resumed in **Table 1**.

In the present work, we include recently obtained data in our laboratory of a prospective comparative multicenter study to evaluate the production of IGFBPs according to liver fibrosis grade in patients with CHC. We provide a valuable and innovative approach to the analysis of IGFBPs as a group of proteins with important potential for improving diagnosis and maybe soon can be used as novel noninvasive biomarkers for liver fibrosis.

Even advanced stages of liver fibrosis have been described as reversible, stimulating considerable research to identify molecules for the development of antifibrotic therapies [35, 36].

IGFBPs are produced in the liver, but there is little evidence of their participation in the process of liver damage in humans. Their study can further improve the knowledge of liver fibrosis pathophysiology and enable the identification of therapeutic targets.

The aim of the present study was to measure the serum concentrations of the different IGFBPs in patients with CHC and analyze them according to the grade of fibrosis grade.

Protein	Production	IGF-dependent functions	IGF-independent functions	Participation in liver	Ref.
IGFBP-1	Liver Kidney Endometrium Amniotic fluid Fetal plasma	Modulates cell growth, differentiation, and metabolism	Proliferation, migration, and apoptosis	↑ Hepatic cirrhosis ↑ F3-F4 in NAFLD	[19]
IGFBP-2	CNS Liver Heart Kidney Prostate Adipocytes	Promotes the bioavailability of IGF to its ligands	Proliferation It binds with TGF-β	Unknown	[33]
IGFBP-3	Liver	Form a ternary complex with IGF and acid-labile subunit (90%)	Survival Activation of MAPK in pulmonary fibrosis Interaction with TGF-β	↓ Cirrhosis, and HCC	[26]
IGFBP-4	Liver Heart Bone Ovary Prostate Kidney	Inhibits angiogenesis Regulates bone formation	Tumor processes and in reproduction biology	Possible role in experimental liver regeneration	[29, 34]
IGFBP-5	Liver Bone Lung Testicle Ovary Uterus Placenta	Form a ternary complex with IGF and acid-labile subunit Inhibits and promotes tumor growth	Inhibits the actions of TNF-α Inhibits and promotes tumor growth proliferation	↑Experimental Fibrosis	[30, 31]
IGFBP-6	Liver Lung Intestine CSN	Inhibits the actions of the IGF-II	Promotes the migration of cancer cell lines Inhibition of angiogenesis	Unknown	[22, 32]
IGFBP-7	Liver	Cell adhesion in cancer cells	Cell proliferation, differentiation, adhesion, senescence, apoptosis, and angiogenesis. Tumoral suppressor Mutual regulation with TGF-β	↓HCC ↑ Experimental and clinical fibrosis	[27, 28]

CNS: Central nervous system, HCC: Hepatocellular carcinoma, F3-F4: advanced stage of fibrosis, ↑ up-regulation and ↓ down-regulation.

Table 1.
Proteins of the IGF system, IGFBPS production, functions, and their regulation in related liver pathologies.

5. Methods and patients for the study of IGFBPs in chronic hepatitis C

A prospective, cross-sectional, observational study was conducted. It included patients seen at the General Hospital of Mexico, University Hospital of Autonomous University of Nuevo Leon, and the National Institute of Medical Sciences and Nutrition, within the time frame of January 2011 to December 2015. The patients were treatment-naïve or untreated, and their grades of fibrosis were evaluated through the FibroTest and FibroScan methods. According to fibrosis grade, the patients were divided into four groups: F0, F1-F2, F3, and F4. Given the small number of patients with stages F1 and F2, they were combined as a single group (n = 25). Patients with at-risk alcohol consumption (AUDIT < 8) and whose fibrosis grade was not determined using the same diagnostic methods stated above were excluded. The control group was made up of healthy subjects, defined as persons that were not at-risk drinkers (AUDIT < 8) and had negative serology for hepatitis A, B, and C viruses (n = 160).

All participants signed statements of informed consent and the study protocol followed the ethics guidelines of the 1975 Declaration of Helsinki. Blood samples (10 mL) were taken from all participants. The serum was separated and stored at −80°C until its use. The anthropometric variables obtained for each study subject were: sex, age, height (measured in centimeters with a stadiometer), weight (measured in kilograms with a manual scale), and body mass index (BMI) (kilograms/meters^2; weight/height^2 formula). The following biochemical tests were performed on all the study subjects: total bilirubin, direct bilirubin, aspartate aminotransferase (AST), and alanine aminotransferase (ALT). A detailed clinical history was carried out for each patient, through which the presence of clinical data of liver damage was intentionally evaluated. IGFBP determination was carried out through multiple suspension array technology (Millipore®). The use of antibodies made it possible to study the concentration of a variable number of proteins in a single serum sample. Thus, seven proteins were analyzed in a single assay, reducing intra-assay and inter-assay error, %CV of <10 and of <15 for intra- and inter-assay, respectively, without cross-reactivity. The HIGFBMAG-53 K07 kit was employed. The data were acquired utilizing Luminex200 MAGPX® Systems equipment (series number 10294005), following the supplier's specifications. The sensitivity of the minimum and maximum detection values for each protein was obtained using Luminex XPONENT software. The continuous variables were described as mean ± standard deviation and the qualitative variables as absolute and relative frequencies (percentages). The qualitative variables were analyzed using the chi-square test and ANOVA test, orthogonal analyses, and Spearman correlation was used for the quantitative variables. Statistical significance was set at $p < 0.05$. Logistic regression analysis with advanced fibrosis stage as the dependent variable was applied. Receiver operating curves (ROCs) were made. Statistical analysis was carried out using the SPSS version 22 program.

6. Clinical determinations

Demographic analysis showed the predominance of women in the group of CHC; furthermore, the age mean was 50 years in CHC in comparison with the mean of 37 years in CT. Nevertheless, body mass index (BMI) did not show differences in both groups of study. Liver function tests that include bilirubin and transaminases (AST and ALT) showed evident and significant increment of values that reflect the liver dysfunction in CHC patients (**Table 1**).

A total of 120 patients diagnosed with chronic hepatitis C (CHC) were included in the study. Many of the patients were women. All the patients were untreated and did not drink alcohol. The control population was made up of 165 healthy subjects with negative viral panels and no at-risk alcohol consumption (**Table 2**).

6.1 Serum determination of IGFBP proteins

As was previously mentioned, the multiple suspension arrangement (Luminex) was used to quantify the levels IGFBP-1 to IGFBP-7 proteins, both in serum of patients with chronic liver disease and in CT. As we expected, a differential regulation of IGFBPs through the different stages of fibrosis in CHC was observed.

6.1.1 IGFBP-1 to IGFBP-7 quantification

IGFBP-1 concentration (ng/mL) was higher in patients compared with controls (1.35 ± 0.26 and 0.65 ± 0.12, respectively, p = 0.02), as were the IGFBP-2 values (16.26 ± 3.81 vs. 3.91 ± 0.35, p = 0.002). IGFBP-3 had the highest concentrations of all the IGFBPs, with a tendency to be lower in patients (778 ± 36) than in controls (878 ± 40, p = 0.066). IGFBP-4 concentrations were higher in patients than in

	CHC (120)	CT (165)	P
Gender n (%)			
Men	25 (29)	138 (89)	<0.001
Women	95 (71)	27 (11)	
Age (years)	51 ± 10	37 ± 9	<0.001
BMI (Kg/m^2)	27 ± 4	28 ± 4	0.464
Total Bilirubin (mg/dl)	1.37 ± 0.22	0.78 ± 0.03	<0.001
Direct Bilirubin (mg/dl)	1.21 ± 0.16	0.68 ± 0.03	<0.001
AST (UI/I)	84 ± 7	30 ± 1	<0.001
ALT (UI/I)	90 ± 6	28 ± 2	<0.001

AST, aspartate amine transferase; ALT, alanine anime transferase. Data are expressed as mean ± standard deviation.

Table 2.
Demographic data of study groups.

IGFBP (ng/mL)	F0 (35)	F1–F2 (11–14)	F3 (21)	F4 (39)	CT (165)	p
1	0.9 ± 0.5	1.5 ± 0.5	1 ± 0.5	1.4 ± 0.5	0.65 ± 0.12	NS
2	8.8 ± 8.4	10 ± 5	26 ± 9	18 ± 7	3.9 ± 3.5	F0vs.CT* F1-F2vs.CT* F3vs.CT† F4vs.CT†
3	695 ± 202	620 ± 350	844 ± 304	756 ± 391	878 ± 406	NS
4	25 ± 17	88 ± 76	37 ± 30	77 ± 29	21 ± 19	F1-F2vs.CT* F3vs.CT* F4vs.CT†
5	97 ± 71	237 ± 186	107 ± 36	324 ± 292	241 ± 118	F4vs.CT* F0vs.F4† F1-F2vs.F3†
6	136 ± 53	112 ± 68	168 ± 81	126 ± 59	122 ± 42	NS
7	20 ± 10	42 ± 30	91 ± 23	60 ± 42	33 ± 31	F3vs.CT† F4vs.CT† F0vs.F3† F0vs.F4* F1-F2vs.F3* F3vs.F4*

*Data are expressed as mean ± standard error (SE). *p < 0.05; † p < 0.005.*

Table 3.
Concentration of IGFBP 1 to 7 and fibrosis stages in patients and control groups.

controls (59 ± 14 vs. 21 ± 1.9, p = 0.008). IGFBP-5 values were similar between patients and controls (251 ± 26 vs. 241 ± 21, p = 0.786), as were IGFBP-6 concentrations (131 ± 6.6 vs. 122 ± 4.2, p = 0.244). IGFBP-7 concentrations were higher in patients (57 ± 4.4), compared with controls (33 ± 3.1) (p < 0.001).

6.1.2 Fibrosis stage and IGFBP analyses

Patients were classified according to 2 noninvasive methods for staging fibrosis: FibroTest and FibroScan. The 120 patients were divided into the following groups: F0 (n = 35), F1–F2 (n = 11–n = 14), F3 (n = 21), and F4 (n = 39). Significant differences were found for IGFBP-2, IGFBP-4, IGFBP-5, and IGFBP-7 (**Table 3**). The differences were mainly between fibrosis grade and the control group for IGFBP-2 and IGFBP 4. IGFBP-2, IGFBP-4, IGFBP-5, and IGFBP-7 concentrations correlated with the grade of fibrosis. There was an association between IGFBP-2 and fibrosis grade (**Figure 1A**), with an r of 0.263 (p = 0.001). IGFBP-4 was increased in F1–F2, F3, and F4, about the control subjects (**Figure 1B**). The correlation of IGFBP-4 with fibrosis grade produced an r of 0.228, (p = 0.003). According to fibrosis grade, there were significant differences between F0 vs. F4 (p < 0.001) and F1-F2 vs. F3 (p < 0.001) in the IGFBP-5 results (**Figure 2A**). We observed an oscillating pattern, given that stages F1–F2 and F4 had the highest concentrations.

There was a 2-fold greater increase in IGFBP-7 concentrations in patients, compared with controls. Upon fibrosis grade evaluation, we found a gradual increase in the concentration of that protein (**Figure 2B**), obtaining significant differences between F0 vs. F3 (p < 0.001), F0 vs. F4 (p < 0.001), F1–F2 vs. F3 (p = 0.002), and F3 vs. F4 (p = 0.005) (**Figure 2B**). The correlation of IGFBP-7 with fibrosis grade

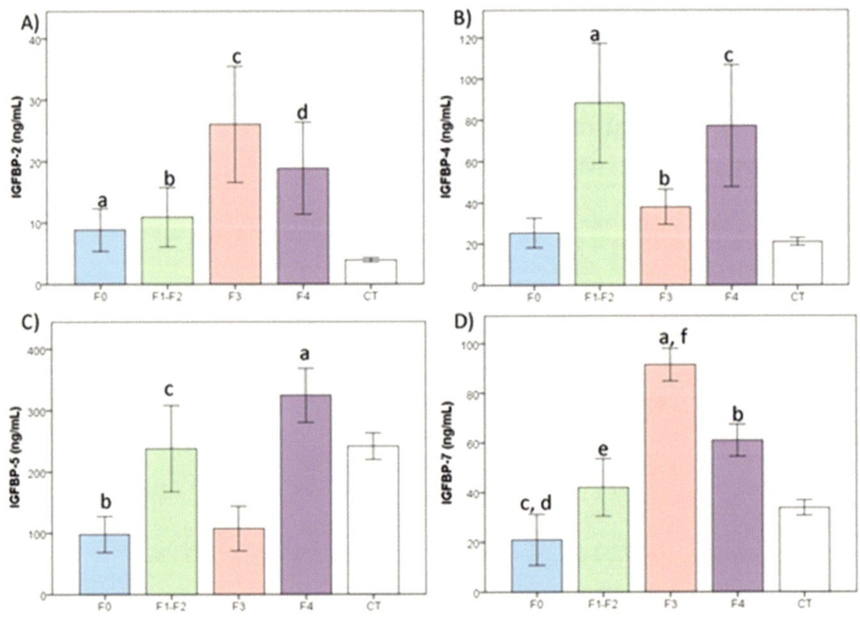

Figure 1.
IGFBP production in different fibrosis stages of CHC compared with healthy individuals. The concentration of IGFBPs (ng/mL) was determined at initial (F0), middle (F1–F2), and severe (F3 and F4) fibrosis stages in CHC and healthy individuals. (A) IGFBP-2 differences: a = F0vs CT (p = 0.002), b = F1–F2 vs. CT (p = 0.01), c = F3 vs. CT (p = 0.001), d = F4 vs. CT (p = 0.001). (B) IGFBP-4 differences: concentrations a = F1–F2 vs. CT (p = 0.002), b = F3 vs. CT (p = 0.008) and c = F4 vs. CT (p = 0.001). (C) IGFBP-5 differences: concentrations a = F4 vs. CT (p = 0.007), b = F0 vs. F4 (p < 0.001), c = F1–F2 vs. F3 (p < 0.001). (D) IGFBP-7 differences: concentrations a = F3 vs. CT (p = 0.001), b = F4 vs. CT (p < 0.001), c = F0 vs. F3 (p < 0.001), d = F0 vs. F4 (p = 0.008), e = F1–F2 vs. F3 (p = 0.002) and f = F3 vs. F4 (p = 0.005). Data are expressed as mean ± standard error (SE).

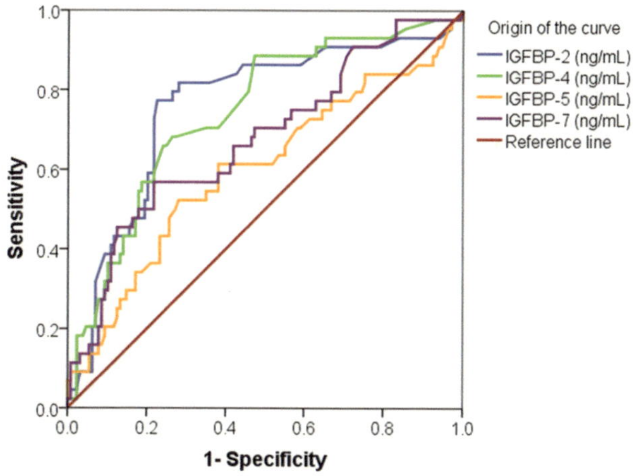

Figure 2.
ROC curve of the concentration of IGFBP-2, -4, -5, and -7 in patients with F4.

produced a statistically significant r of 0.384 ($p = 0.001$), indicating that IGFBP-7 was associated with the grade of fibrosis, signifying that it could be a serologic biomarker for liver fibrosis.

Moreover, our study provides for first time completed screening of seven IGFBPs and their serum concentration in the initial, middle, and severe fibrosis stages. For IGFBP-1, slight differences in middle and severe stages and CT were found, whereas nonsignificant differences were observed for de IGFBP-3, and -6 among F0, F1–F2, F3, F4, and CT classifications. However, evident variations were observed for IGFBP-2 and -4 according to the fibrosis degrees and CT group. (**Table 3**). The most evident concentration changes were observed in IGFBP-7, where the statistical analysis revealed a correlation in the fibrosis degrees and their production (**Table 3**).

6.1.3 Sensitivity and specificity of IGFBPs in severe fibrosis stage

Additionally, we performed calculation of the area under the receiver operating characteristic curve (AUROC) using the severe stage as a reference parameter with the aim to determine the sensitivity and specificity of IGFBP-2, -4, -5, and -7 with F4 stage (**Figure 2** and **Table 4**). The results showed that the value of area under the curve for IGFBP-2 was 0.760 ($p < 0.001$; 95% CI, 0.672–0.847); whereas in IGFBP-4 was 0.744 ($p < 0.001$; 95% CI, 0.659–0.828), IGFBP-5 was 0.600 ($p = 0.049$; 95% CI, 0.496–0.703), and for IGFBP-7 was 0.674 ($p = 0.001$; 95% CI, 0.579–0.770) (**Table 4**). Based on the AUROC interpretation, where the

Protein	Area	95%CI		p
		Lower limit	Upper limit	
IGFBP-2 (ng/mL)	0.760	0.672	0.847	0.000
IGFBP-4 (ng/mL)	0.744	0.659	0.828	0.000
IGFBP-5 (ng/mL)	0.600	0.496	0.703	0.049
IGFBP-7 (ng/mL)	0.674	0.579	0.770	0.001

Table 4.
Evaluation of the area under the ROC curve of IGFBP-2, -4, -5, and -7 in patients with severe fibrosis degree (F4).

values take more significance when they are close to the unit and with p value, we observed that the degree of predictive significance indicator of these proteins is: IGFBP2 < IGFBP-4 < IGFBP-7 < IGFBP-5.

7. Discussion

Our study is the first to quantify seven IGFBPs in patients with hepatitis C virus (HCV) and associate those protein levels with fibrosis grade. Different studies consider IGFBP-1 as an insulin-sensitive protein that participates in the development of metabolic diseases, such as insulin-resistance or metabolic syndrome, in patients with or without liver disease. Some authors have reported elevated levels of IGFBP-1 expression [37], whereas others have found low levels [38, 39]. Because of findings of its increased expression, IGFBP-1 has been identified as a possible biomarker for alcoholic liver disease (ALD). Controversial results have been reported in relation to NAFLD. A decrease in serum concentrations due to interaction with insulin was described [40, 41], but Hagström et al. reported elevated values, with higher concentrations in patients with advanced fibrosis [19]. High concentrations have also been associated with hepatocellular carcinoma, albeit the role of that protein is still contradictory [37, 42]. In our study, IGFBP-1 concentrations were higher in subjects with CHC, but no differences were found in relation to fibrosis grade. However, studies on patients with liver cirrhosis of different etiologies (hepatitis C, hepatitis B, NAFLD, ALD, and autoimmune hepatitis) have shown that IGFBP-1 increases [19, 43] and is higher in advanced fibrosis (F3 and F4) [19].

IGFBP-2 has been suggested as a biomarker for metabolic diseases, such as diabetes and insulin resistance [33]. In our study, IGFBP-2 concentrations were until 6-fold higher in patients, compared with controls. In accordance with fibrosis grade, there was also a gradual increase in IGFBP-2 concentration, but with no statistically significant differences between fibrosis stages, suggesting that IGFBP-2 participates in liver damage and the development of fibrosis caused by HCV. Our results concur with those reported for idiopathic pulmonary fibrosis, in which high levels of IGFBP-2 were determined [44].

Additionally, in this work, we can determine for first time the evaluation of the specificity and sensibility of the seven IGFBPs. Interestingly, IGFBP-2 showed higher area values (AUROC) in F4 and thus can be considered as the best predictive IGFBP protein indicator in severe fibrosis stage followed by -4, -7 and -5.

IGFBP-3 had higher concentration levels than those of the other six IGFBPs. Nevertheless, the concentrations showed a tendency to be lower in patients than in controls. IGFBP-3 has been the most widely studied protein because of its high affinity for IGF-I. It has been described as a biomarker for liver dysfunction classified with the Child-Pugh scale, with a lower concentration in patients with Child-Pugh class C [45]. Since 1995, many studies have been conducted on IGFBPs in patients with liver cirrhosis due to different causes. Results have shown a decrease in IGFBP-3 concentrations and an increase in IGF-I [46, 47]. IGFBPs are also thought to be associated with a high risk for liver cancer [48] and with poor prognosis [26]. Aleem et al. concluded that IGFBP-3 is superior to IGF-I and IGF-II for predicting the development of hepatocellular carcinoma in patients with cirrhosis caused by HCV [49], due to viral protein interaction that alters the IGF axis and the subsequent progression to liver cancer [50].

Miller et al. described the serum proteome of NAFLD, reporting increased IGFBP-3, compared with control subjects. They then analyzed fibrosis grade and severity and found that IGFBP-3 was able to distinguish between different disease stages [51]. In 2017, Chishima et al. studied the GH/IGF-I/IGFBP-3 axis in patients with NAFLD and CHC and the relation to the histologic severity of NAFLD. IGFBP-3 levels were lower in patients with cirrhosis caused by NAFLD, whereas the levels did not decrease according to fibrosis grade in patients with HCV-induced chronic liver disease [46]. Our results concurred with those of that study.

Cirrhosis alters IGF-I production and suppresses protein metabolism. In studies on children with end-stage liver disease (ESLD) who underwent liver transplantation, the authors concluded that their results partially explained the failure to growth and the reduced number of functioning hepatocytes in patients with ESLD [52].

IGFBP-4 has been associated with the progression of lung cancer, finding high expression of that protein in lung tissue, and showing a decrease in survival [53]. In our study, IGFBP-4 concentration was 2-fold higher in patients, compared with controls, and behavior fluctuated in relation to fibrosis grade, with no statistically significant differences. In a study on patients with ESLD, no differences in IGFBP-4 were found upon comparison before and after liver transplantation [52]. In another study on cirrhotic patients and controls, there were no differences in IGFBP-4 when measured by the Western ligand blot technique [54]. Experimental studies have shown a regulation of the increase of that protein, along with IGFBP-1 and IGF-I, by AMPc, IL-6, IL-1β, and TNF-α [55, 56].

IGFBP-5 has been studied in animal models of progressive intrahepatic cholestasis, suggesting that it plays a possible role in the pathogenesis of chronic cholangiopathy. The same authors reported that IGFBP-5, in human stellate cells (LX-2), increased pro-fibrotic marker expression, and concluded that IGFBP-5 participates in liver fibrosis progression [30]. In our study, IGFBP-5 concentrations were similar between patients and controls. However, upon classifying them by fibrosis grade, we found differences in F0 vs. F4 and F1–F2 vs. F3. These findings concur with the results reported by Colak et al. who showed that IGFBP-5 played an important role in many pathophysiologic stages of liver fibrosis [57]. One of the functions of IGFBP-5 was the trans-differentiation of HSCs into myofibroblasts, improving the survival of those cells through anti-apoptotic effects on the activated HSCs, increasing collagen Iα1, TIMP-1, and MMP-1profibrotic gene expression.

It is known that IGFBP-6 can induce chemotaxis in T cells and monocytes, but not in B cells. It also increases oxidative stress and may be a late amplifier of neutrophil activation [58]. However, there have been few studies conducted on IGFBP-6 in liver diseases. In our study, IGFBP-6 concentrations were the same in patients and controls, and we found a tendency for concentrations to increase with the increase in fibrosis grade. IGFBP-6 has been described to be affected by HCV proteins and to participate in the progression to liver cancer [50, 59].

Finally, different studies demonstrate that IGFBP-7 (IGFBPrP1) contributes to liver fibrogenesis [27, 60, 61]. In our study, we found a significant increase in patients with liver disease. Likewise, we observed a gradual increase according to fibrosis grade. It was higher in F3, indicating that it could be a serum biomarker for liver fibrosis. IGFBP-7 has been widely studied in experimental models of liver fibrosis for identifying the mechanisms involved in the activation of HSCs and the signaling pathways, the result of which induces fibrosis. IGFBP-7 was inhibited in rat HSCs, inducing apoptosis in activated HSCs, and as a result, ameliorating liver fibrogenesis [61]. IGFBP-7 has also been shown to attenuate liver fibrosis through the regulation of MMPs/TIMPs in mice [62]. IGFBPrP1 contributed to the development of liver fibrosis in fibrotic and cirrhotic tissue biopsy samples and may be a novel molecule involved in the progression of liver fibrogenesis [28]. Studies conducted in vitro found that IGFBPrP1 induced liver fibrosis by means of HSC activation and hepatocyte apoptosis through the Smad 2/3 signaling pathway [27]. In addition, it acted as an initiator of liver fibrosis by inducing inflammation, HSC activation, and ECM protein deposit through the ERK1/2 pathway [63]. IGFBPrP1 has also been shown to promote fibrosis, by enhancing the TGF-β1 expression that it triggered, and the Egr1, PTEN, Hhip, MAP2K2 (MEK2), and MAPK3 (ERK1) genes were identified as candidates for the hepatic fibrosis-related pathway induced by IGFBPrP1 [60]. Mutual IGFBPrP1 and TGF-β1 regulation has been found that probably accelerates liver fibrosis progression [64]. IGFBPrP1 inhibition attenuates fibrosis by reestablishing the MMP2/TIMP2 and MMP9/TIMP1 balance concomitantly with the inhibition of HSC activation, low TGF-β1 expression, and ECM degradation [62]. Previous results, together with ours, show that IGFBP-7 is a molecule that can be diagnostically useful and a possible therapeutic target for liver fibrosis.

Currently, there are available treatment regiments against hepatitis C; in general, these drugs have as specific targets viral proteins (e. g. NS3/4A, NS5A, and NS5B) inhibiting their replication. The ratio of efficacy of different combinations of drugs can reach until 95% of efficiency [65, 66]. Regarding the action of these drugs and liver fibrosis, it has been reported that peginterferon and/or ribavirin, daclatasvir, sofosbuvir, and simeprevir can cause regression of liver fibrosis [67]. The specific molecular events induced by the administration of these drugs are not very well understood. However, it has been observed that the liver parenchymal injury and hepatocyte death are associated with the host's inflammatory response and reactive oxygen species promoted by virus proteins [68, 69], whereby the elimination of viral load abrogates the subsequent liver damage. Nevertheless, the molecular mechanisms triggered by the pharmacological therapy in the IGF system are not evaluated until now; it is possible that tissue fibrosis reversion can be orchestrated by IGF elements such as the IGFBPs. Thus, the study of these proteins could have beneficial implication for diagnosis and as well as complementary target to improve the liver regeneration.

8. Conclusion

We found higher serum concentrations of IGFBP-2, IGFBP-4, IGFBP-5, and IGFBP-7 in patients with CHC, and in accordance with fibrosis grade, IGFBP-2, IGFBP-4, and IGFBP-7 are associated with severe fibrosis. Based on our study, we strongly suggest the possibility that IGFBPs participate in ECM protein modulation and reuptake and regulate the progression of chronic liver disease and development of liver fibrosis. Therefore, we believe that IGF binding proteins play an important role in chronic hepatitis C and can be serum marker candidates for liver fibrosis.

Acknowledgements

This work was supported by CONACyT Grant Number SALUD-2016-272579, PAPIIT- UNAM TA200515 and postdoctoral fellowship DGAPA-UNAM.

Conflict of interest

The authors have no conflict of interest or financial conflict with any organization or entity.

Author details

Dorothy Rosique-Oramas[1], Moisés Martínez-Castillo[1], Carolina Guzman[1], José Luis Pérez Hernández[3], Jacqueline Cordova-Gallardo[5], Luis Very-Pineda[1], Fatima Higuera-De La Tijera[3], Daniel Santana-Vargas[3], Eduardo Montalvo-Jave[3], Francisco Sanchez-Avila[2], Paula Cordero-Perez[4], Linda Muñoz-Espinosa[4], David Kershenobich[1,2] and Gabriela Gutiérrez-Reyes[1]*

1 HIPAM Laboratory, Experimental Medicine Unit, School of Medicine, National Autonomous University of Mexico, Mexico City, México

2 National Institute of Medical Sciences and Nutrition "Salvador Zubirán", Mexico City, México

3 General Hospital of Mexico "Dr. Eduardo Liceaga", Mexico City, México

4 University Hospital "Dr. José Eleuterio González", Autonomous University of Nuevo Leon, Monterrey, México

5 General Hospital "Dr. Manuel Gea González", Mexico City, México

*Address all correspondence to: gabgurey@yahoo.com.mx

References

[1] Rockey DC, Bell PD, Hill JA. Fibrosis—A common pathway to organ injury and failure. The New England Journal of Medicine. 2015;**373**(1):96. Epub: 2015/06/02

[2] Pellicoro A, Ramachandran P, Iredale JP, Fallowfield JA. Liver fibrosis and repair: Immune regulation of wound healing in a solid organ. Nature Reviews. Immunology. 2014;**14**(3):181-194. Epub: 2014/02/26

[3] Elpek GO. Cellular and molecular mechanisms in the pathogenesis of liver fibrosis: An update. World Journal of Gastroenterology. 2014;**20**(23): 7260-7276. Epub: 2014/06/27

[4] Seki E, Brenner DA. Recent advancement of molecular mechanisms of liver fibrosis. Journal of Hepato-Biliary-Pancreatic Sciences. 2015;**22**(7):512-518. Epub: 2015/04/15

[5] Schuppan D, Ashfaq-Khan M, Yang AT, Kim YO. Liver fibrosis: Direct antifibrotic agents and targeted therapies. Matrix Biology : Journal of the International Society for Matrix Biology. 2018;**68-69**:435-451. Epub: 2018/04/16

[6] Trivedi HD, Lin SC, Lau DYT. Noninvasive assessment of fibrosis regression in hepatitis C virus sustained virologic responders. Gastroenterology & Hepatology. 2017;**13**(10):587-595. Epub: 2018/02/03

[7] Zoubek ME, Trautwein C, Strnad P. Reversal of liver fibrosis: From fiction to reality. Best Practice & Research. Clinical Gastroenterology. 2017;**31**(2):129-141. Epub: 2017/06/19

[8] Nallagangula KS, Nagaraj SK, Venkataswamy L, Chandrappa M. Liver fibrosis: A compilation on the biomarkers status and their significance during disease progression. Future Science OA. 2018;**4**(1):FSO250. Epub: 2017/12/20

[9] Bedossa P, Carrat F. Liver biopsy: The best, not the gold standard. Journal of Hepatology. 2009;**50**(1):1-3. Epub: 2008/11/20

[10] Pokora A, Kiciak S, Tomasiewicz K. Assessing the consistency of liver fibrosis results obtained through biopsy and transient elastography in patients suffering from chronic hepatitis C. Clinical and Experimental Hepatology. 2016;**2**(3):109-111. Epub: 2017/09/01

[11] Trabut JB, Plat A, Thepot V, Fontaine H, Vallet-Pichard A, Nalpas B, et al. Influence of liver biopsy on abstinence in alcohol-dependent patients. Alcohol and Alcoholism. 2008;**43**(5):559-563. Epub: 2008/07/16

[12] Oliveri F, Coco B, Ciccorossi P, Colombatto P, Romagnoli V, Cherubini B, et al. Liver stiffness in the hepatitis B virus carrier: A non-invasive marker of liver disease influenced by the pattern of transaminases. World Journal of Gastroenterology. 2008;**14**(40): 6154-6162. Epub: 2008/11/06

[13] de Ledinghen V, Vergniol J, Gonzalez C, Foucher J, Maury E, Chemineau L, et al. Screening for liver fibrosis by using FibroScan((R)) and FibroTest in patients with diabetes. Digestive and Liver Disease: Official Journal of the Italian Society of Gastroenterology and the Italian Association for the Study of the Liver. 2012;**44**(5):413-418. Epub: 2012/01/31

[14] Nguyen-Khac E, Thiele M, Voican C, Nahon P, Moreno C, Boursier J, et al. Non-invasive diagnosis of liver fibrosis in patients with alcohol-related liver disease by transient elastography: An individual patient data meta-analysis.

The Lancet Gastroenterology & Hepatology. 2018;**3**(9):614-625. Epub: 2018/07/10

[15] van Katwyk S, Coyle D, Cooper C, Pussegoda K, Cameron C, Skidmore B, et al. Transient elastography for the diagnosis of liver fibrosis: A systematic review of economic evaluations. Liver International: Official Journal of the International Association for the Study of the Liver. 2017;**37**(6):851-861. Epub: 2016/10/25

[16] Weiss J, Rau M, Meertens J, Hering I, Reichert L, Kudlich T, et al. Feasibility of liver stiffness measurement in morbidly obese patients undergoing bariatric surgery using XL probe. Scandinavian Journal of Gastroenterology. 2016;**51**(10):1263-1268

[17] Papastergiou V, Tsochatzis E, Burroughs AK. Non-invasive assessment of liver fibrosis. Annals of Gastroenterology. 2012;**25**(3):218-231. Epub: 2012/01/01

[18] Shaheen AA, Wan AF, Myers RP. FibroTest and FibroScan for the prediction of hepatitis C-related fibrosis: A systematic review of diagnostic test accuracy. The American Journal of Gastroenterology. 2007;**102**(11): 2589-2600. Epub: 2007/09/14

[19] Hagstrom H, Stal P, Hultcrantz R, Brismar K, Ansurudeen I. IGFBP-1 and IGF-I as markers for advanced fibrosis in NAFLD—A pilot study. Scandinavian Journal of Gastroenterology. 2017;**52**(12):1427-1434. Epub: 2017/09/21

[20] Foulstone E, Prince S, Zaccheo O, Burns JL, Harper J, Jacobs C, et al. Insulin-like growth factor ligands, receptors, and binding proteins in cancer. Journal of Pathology. 2005;**205**(2):145-153

[21] Pollak MN. Insulin, insulin-like growth factors, insulin resistance, and neoplasia. American Journal of Clinical Nutrition. 2007;**86**(3):820s-822s

[22] Pollak M. Insulin and insulin-like growth factor signalling in neoplasia. Nature Reviews. Cancer. 2008;**8**(12):915-928

[23] Firth SM, Baxter RC. Cellular actions of the insulin-like growth factor binding proteins. Endocrine Reviews. 2002;**23**(6):824-854. Epub: 2002/12/06

[24] Hwa V, Oh Y, Rosenfeld RG. The insulin-like growth factor-binding protein (IGFBP) superfamily. Endocrine Reviews. 1999;**20**(6):761-787

[25] Boers W, Aarrass S, Linthorst C, Pinzani M, Elferink RO, Bosma P. Transcriptional profiling reveals novel markers of liver fibrogenesis—Gremlin and insulin-like growth factor-binding proteins. Journal of Biological Chemistry. 2006;**281**(24):16289-16295

[26] Yan JJ, Yang XZ, Li L, Liu PT, Wu HH, Liu ZN, et al. Low expression levels of insulin-like growth factor binding protein-3 are correlated with poor prognosis for patients with hepatocellular carcinoma. Oncology Letters. 2017;**13**(5):3395-3402

[27] Zhang Y, Zhang QQ, Guo XH, Zhang HY, Liu LX. IGFBPrP1 induces liver fibrosis by inducing hepatic stellate cell activation and hepatocyte apoptosis via Smad2/3 signaling. World Journal of Gastroenterology. 2014;**20**(21):6523-6533

[28] Guo XH, Liu LX, Zhang HY, Zhang QQ, Li Y, Tian XX, et al. Insulin-like growth factor binding protein-related protein 1 contributes to hepatic fibrogenesis. Journal of Digestive Diseases. 2014;**15**(4):202-210

[29] Wright RJ, Holly JMP, Galea R, Brincat M, Mason HD. Insulin-like growth factor (IGF)-independent effects of IGF binding protein-4 on

human granulosa cell steroidogenesis. Biology of Reproduction. 2002;**67**(3):776-781

[30] Sokolovic A, Sokolovic M, Boers W, Elferink RP, Bosma PJ. Insulin-like growth factor binding protein 5 enhances survival of LX2 human hepatic stellate cells. Fibrogenesis & Tissue Repair. 2010;**3**:3. Epub: 2010/02/19

[31] Hwang JR, Huh JH, Lee Y, Lee SI, Rho SB, Lee JH. Insulin-like growth factor-binding protein-5 (IGFBP-5) inhibits TNF-alpha-induced NF-kappa B activity by binding to TNFR1. Biochemical and Biophysical Research Communications. 2011;**405**(4):545-551

[32] Fu P, Thompson JA, Bach LA. Promotion of cancer cell migration—An insulin-like growth factor (IGF)-independent action of IGF-binding protein-6. Journal of Biological Chemistry. 2007;**282**(31):22298-22306

[33] Shin M, Kang HS, Park JH, Bae JH, Song DK, Im SS. Recent insights into insulin-like growth factor binding protein 2 transcriptional regulation. Endocrinology and Metabolism-ENM. 2017;**32**(1):11-17

[34] Demori I, Balocco S, Voci A, Fugassa E. Increased insulin-like growth factor binding protein-4 expression after partial hepatectomy in the rat. American Journal of Physiology. Gastrointestinal and Liver Physiology. 2000;**278**(3):G384-G389. Epub: 2000/03/11

[35] Friedman SL, Bansal MB. Reversal of hepatic fibrosis—Fact or fantasy? Hepatology. 2006;**43**(2):S82-SS8

[36] Ellis EL, Mann DA. Clinical evidence for the regression of liver fibrosis. Journal of Hepatology. 2012;**56**(5):1171-1180

[37] Hwang DL, Huang SP, Lan WS, Lee PDK. Elevated insulin, proinsulin and insulin-like growth factor-binding protein-1 in liver disease. Growth Hormone & IGF Research. 2003;**13**(6):316-321

[38] Alberstein M, Zornitzki T, Zick Y, Knobler H. Hepatitis C core protein impairs insulin downstream signalling and regulatory role of IGFBP-1 expression. Journal of Viral Hepatitis. 2012;**19**(1):65-71

[39] Heald AH, Cruickshank JK, Riste LK, Cade JE, Anderson S, Greenhalgh A, et al. Close relation of fasting insulin-like growth factor binding protein-1 (IGFBP-1) with glucose tolerance and cardiovascular risk in two populations. Diabetologia. 2001;**44**(3):333-339

[40] Petaja EM, Zhou Y, Havana M, Hakkarainen A, Lundbom N, Ihalainen J, et al. Phosphorylated IGFBP-1 as a non-invasive predictor of liver fat in NAFLD. Scientific Reports. 2016;**6**:24740. Epub: 2016/04/20

[41] Graffigna MN, Belli SH, de Larranaga G, Fainboim H, Estepo C, Peres S, et al. Insulin-like growth factor-binding protein-1: A new biochemical marker of nonalcoholic fatty liver disease? [La proteina transportadora del factor de crecimiento insulinico tipo 1: Un nuevo marcador para la enfermedad hepatica grasa no alcoholica?]. Acta Gastroenterologica Latinoamericana. 2009;**39**(1):30-37. Epub: 2009/05/05

[42] Dai B, Ruan B, Wu J, Wang J, Shang R, Sun W, et al. Insulin-like growth factor binding protein-1 inhibits cancer cell invasion and is associated with poor prognosis in hepatocellular carcinoma. International Journal of Clinical and Experimental Pathology. 2014;**7**(9):5645-5654. Epub: 2014/10/23

[43] Ormarsdottir S, Ljunggren O, Mallmin H, Olofsson H, Blum WF, Loof L. Circulating levels of insulin-like

growth factors and their binding proteins in patients with chronic liver disease: Lack of correlation with bone mineral density. Liver. 2001;**21**(2): 123-128. Epub: 2001/04/25

[44] Guiot J, Bondue B, Henket M, Corhay JL, Louis R. Raised serum levels of IGFBP-1 and IGFBP-2 in idiopathic pulmonary fibrosis. BMC Pulmonary Medicine. 2016;**16**(1):86. Epub: 2016/05/25

[45] Correa CG, Colombo BD, Ronsoni MF, Silva PESE, Fayad L, Silva TE, et al. Circulating insulin-like growth factor-binding protein 3 as prognostic biomarker in liver cirrhosis. World Journal of Hepatology. 2016;**8**(17):739-748

[46] Chishima S, Kogiso T, Matsushita N, Hashimoto E, Tokushige K. The relationship between the growth hormone/insulin-like growth factor system and the histological features of nonalcoholic fatty liver disease. Internal Medicine. 2017;**56**(5):473-480. Epub: 2017/03/03

[47] Donaghy A, Ross R, Gimson A, Hughes SC, Holly J, Williams R. Growth hormone, insulinlike growth factor-1, and insulinlike growth factor binding proteins 1 and 3 in chronic liver disease. Hepatology. 1995;**21**(3):680-688. Epub: 1995/03/01

[48] Adachi Y, Nojima M, Mori M, Matsunaga Y, Akutsu N, Sasaki S, et al. Insulin-like growth factor-related components and the risk of liver cancer in a nested case-control study. Tumour Biology. 2016;**37**(11):15125-15132. Epub: 2016/09/25

[49] Aleem E, Elshayeb A, Elhabachi N, Mansour AR, Gowily A, Hela A. Serum IGFBP-3 is a more effective predictor than IGF-1 and IGF-2 for the development of hepatocellular carcinoma in patients with chronic HCV infection. Oncology Letters. 2012;**3**(3):704-712. Epub: 2012/06/29

[50] Kasprzak A, Adamek A. The insulin-like growth factor (IGF) signaling axis and hepatitis C virus-associated carcinogenesis (review). International Journal of Oncology. 2012;**41**(6):1919-1931. Epub: 2012/10/19

[51] Miller MH, Walsh SV, Atrih A, Huang JT, Ferguson MA, Dillon JF. Serum proteome of nonalcoholic fatty liver disease: A multimodal approach to discovery of biomarkers of nonalcoholic steatohepatitis. Journal of Gastroenterology and Hepatology. 2014;**29**(10):1839-1847. Epub: 2014/04/23

[52] Schalch DS, Kalayoglu M, Pirsch JD, Yang H, Raslich M, Rajpal S. Serum insulin-like growth factors and their binding proteins in patients with hepatic failure and after liver transplantation. Metabolism. 1998;**47**(2):200-206. Epub: 1998/02/24

[53] Xiao Y, Zhu S, Yin W, Liu XF, Hu Y. IGFBP-4 expression is adversely associated with lung cancer prognosis. Oncology Letters. 2017;**14**(6):6876-6880

[54] Moller S, Juul A, Becker U, Flyvbjerg A, Skakkebaek NE, Henriksen JH. Concentrations, release, and disposal of insulin-like growth-factor (Igf)-binding proteins (Igfbp), Igf-I, and growth-hormone in different vascular beds in patients with cirrhosis. The Journal of Clinical Endocrinology and Metabolism. 1995; **80**(4):1148-1157

[55] Scharf JG, Dombrowski F, Ramadori G. The IGF axis and hepatocarcinogenesis. Molecular Pathology: MP. 2001;**54**(3):138-144. Epub: 2001/05/29

[56] Lelbach A, Scharf JG, Ramadori G. Regulation of insulin-like growth factor-I and of insulin-like growth

factor binding protein-1, -3 and -4 in cocultures of rat hepatocytes and Kupffer cells by interleukin-6. Journal of Hepatology. 2001;**35**(5):558-567. Epub: 2001/11/03

[57] Colak Y, Senates E, Ozturk O, Yilmaz Y, Zemheri E, Yilmaz Enc F, et al. Serum concentrations of human insulin-like growth factor-1 and levels of insulin-like growth factor-binding protein-5 in patients with nonalcoholic fatty liver disease: Association with liver histology. European Journal of Gastroenterology & Hepatology. 2012;**24**(3):255-261. Epub: 2011/12/14

[58] Conese M, D'Oria S, Castellani S, Trotta R, Montemurro P, Liso A. Insulin-like growth factor-6 (IGFBP-6) stimulates neutrophil oxidative burst, degranulation and chemotaxis. Inflammation Research. 2018;**67**(2):107-109

[59] Bach LA, Fu P, Yang ZY. Insulin-like growth factor-binding protein-6 and cancer. Clinical Science. 2013;**124**(3-4):215-229

[60] Guo XH, Zhang HY, Zhang QQ, Li XQ, Liu LX. Screening for and validation of a hepatic fibrosis-related pathway induced by insulin-like growth factor-binding protein-related protein 1. European Journal of Gastroenterology & Hepatology. 2016;**28**(7):762-772

[61] Liu LX, Huang S, Zhang QQ, Liu Y, Zhang DM, Guo XH, et al. Insulin-like growth factor binding protein-7 induces activation and transdifferentiation of hepatic stellate cells in vitro. World Journal of Gastroenterology. 2009;**15**(26):3246-3253. Epub: 2009/07/15

[62] Ren JJ, Huang TJ, Zhang QQ, Zhang HY, Guo XH, Fan HQ, et al. Insulin-like growth factor binding protein related protein 1 knockdown attenuates hepatic fibrosis via the regulation of MMPs/TIMPs in mice. Hepatobiliary & Pancreatic Diseases International. 2018. Epub: 2018/09/24

[63] Guo YR, Zhang Y, Zhang QQ, Guo XH, Zhang HY, Zheng GP, et al. Insulin-like growth factor binding protein-related protein 1 (IGFBPrP1) contributes to liver inflammation and fibrosis via activation of the ERK1/2 pathway. Hepatology International. 2015;**9**(1):130-141

[64] Li XQ, Zhang QQ, Zhang HY, Guo XH, Fan HQ, Liu LX. Interaction between insulin-like growth factor binding protein-related protein 1 and transforming growth factor beta 1 in primary hepatic stellate cells. Hepatobiliary & Pancreatic Diseases International. 2017;**16**(4):395-404

[65] Burstow NJ, Mohamed Z, Gomaa AI, Sonderup MW, Cook NA, Waked I, et al. Hepatitis C treatment: Where are we now? International Journal of General Medicine. 2017;**10**:39-52

[66] Dick TB, Lindberg LS, Ramirez DD, Charlton MR. A clinician's guide to drug-drug interactions with direct-acting antiviral agents for the treatment of hepatitis C viral infection. Hepatology. 2016;**63**(2):634-643

[67] Parola M, Pinzani M. Liver fibrosis: Pathophysiology, pathogenetic targets and clinical issues. Molecular Aspects of Medicine. 2018. Epub: 2018/09/15

[68] Guidotti LG, Chisari FV. Immunobiology and pathogenesis of viral hepatitis. Annual Review of Pathology. 2006;**1**:23-61. Epub: 2007/11/28

[69] Bataller R, Paik YH, Lindquist JN, Lemasters JJ, Brenner DA. Hepatitis C virus core and nonstructural proteins induce fibrogenic effects in hepatic stellate cells. Gastroenterology. 2004;**126**(2):529-540

Chapter 2

Genetics of Biliary Atresia: A Work in Progress for a Disease with an Unavoidable Sequela into Liver Cirrhosis following Failure of Hepatic Portoenterostomy

Consolato M. Sergi

Abstract

The bile duct development may not be fully completed at birth, and this is quite a common event. Moreover, bile formation is immature, and there is a propensity for the neonate to develop cholestasis in the presence of a wide variety of insults that can damage the liver. A biliary atresia is a correctable form of infantile cholangiopathies. The Kasai hepatic portoenterostomy (HPE) is often performed and is successful if it is done at an early stage. However, HPE can fail, and the liver fate is inevitably a cirrhotic change. Biliary atresia is heterogeneous and may result from a combination of genetic factors, vascular, infective or toxic insults with activation of different genetic and immunological pathways. In this chapter, we will review some genes that may be highly relevant to biliary atresia, including not only PKHD1, JAG1, and CFTR, but also GPC1, ADD3 and others. Four genetic loci are considered as predisposition loci in biliary atresia, despite the absence of an etiologic mutation. The rare occurrence of biliary atresia in well-known genetic syndromes seems to suggest coincidental finding, but epigenetic aspects might play a significant role in contributing to the increase of biliary atresia rate.

Keywords: biliary atresia, cirrhosis, kasai failure, genes, bioinformatics

1. Introduction

Biliary atresia (BA) is a necroinflammatory process of the intrahepatic (inside of the liver) and extrahepatic (outside of the liver) biliary system with a various etiologic background. Since the introduction of the yellow card registries in Taiwan in 2002 as a pilot study and then in other countries, the awareness and the proper management of this disease has increased. In the Western countries, BA occurs in about 1:18,000 live births, but the reported incidences vary from 5 to 32 per 10^5 live births [1]. The incidence of BA is highest in Asia and in some countries of the Pacific region comparing to the rest of the world with male infants more often affected than females. The clinical triad includes neonatal jaundice (conjugated hyperbilirubinemia that is considered lasting beyond 2 weeks of postnatal life), acholic (pale) stools and dark urine, and hepatomegaly. The ultrasonography and

IntechOpen

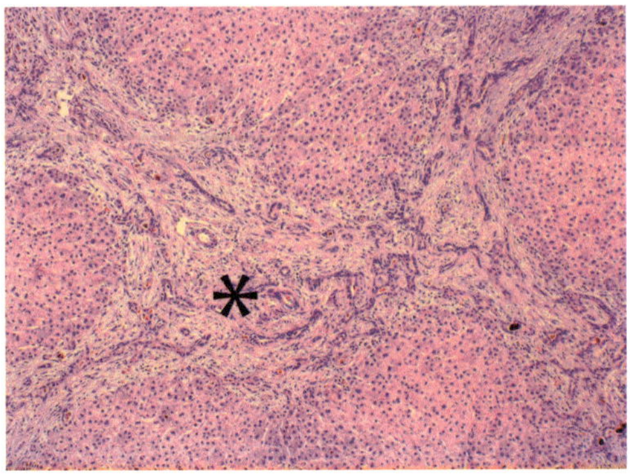

Figure 1.
Biliary atresia with extensive fibrosis and bile duct proliferations (asterisk) (Hematoxylin and eosin staining, x100 original magnification).

the endoscopic retrograde cholangiopancreatography (ERCP) are essential to address the diagnosis, which relies on the microscopic examination. Histologically, BA relies on the inflammatory injury of the intra- and extrahepatic biliary tract with sclerosis, luminal narrowing, and final obliteration of the biliary tree. BA lead to liver cirrhosis, if no treatment is initiated. Also, death can occur within the 2 years of life or first infancy. Although BA is, currently, not known to be hereditary, some families with recurrence of this disease have been reported in the literature. BA requires an immediate shunt to promote the discharge of bilirubin from the progressive accumulation in the liver and Professor Morlo Kasai (1922–2008) invented a technique (Kasai hepatic portoenterostomy or HPE), which is currently in use and the first line of surgical therapy for these patients [2–4]. Subsequently, a liver transplantation may be needed, particularly in infants who underwent to surgery not early in life as it should be. The delay of the surgical hepatic portoenterostomy is still a problem in some regions not only in underdeveloped countries, but even in USA and Canada. Thus, the awareness of this condition is crucial to save lives and money. Liver transplantation may be crucial needed to restore the flow of bile or if liver cirrhotic complications occur (**Figure 1**). Currently, nearly 90% of BA infants survive. The majority of these patients have normal quality of life. Prof. Kasai is considered one of the greatest innovators in the field of pediatric surgery and numerous thousands of babies and their families will be always grateful to him.

2. Bile duct development

The development of the biliary tree is crucial to understand and interpret the categories of neonatal and infantile cholangiopathies. This aspect is particularly important if the patient is a preterm baby or a baby considered small for gestational age [5]. At the 3rd week of the post-ovulatory period, endodermal cells sprout from the primitive foregut at the cranial portion. These cells grow towards a loosely arranged mesoderm. The direction is the *plexus vitellinus* of the embryo. Similarly, a bud arises caudally from the foregut and form the primordium (anlage) of the extrahepatic biliary system [5–8]. After a sub-massive and massive liver necrosis, a ductular reaction is observed in the survived liver tissue. This phenomenon is seen in individuals with fulminant hepatitis and endorses the theory recommending the presence of ordinary progenitor cells that may totally differentiate in bile duct epithelial cells, specifically along the portal vein branches [9]. At the hilum of the liver between the 6th and the 9th week of the postovulatory period, progenitor cells, which are in contact with the mesenchyme that surrounds the primitive portal vein, form first a mono-layered and then later a double-layered cell cords harboring a "slit-like" lumen [5, 10]. This structure is the fundamental (primitive) intrahepatic biliary structure, which has been labeled (bilaminar) "ductal plate." At the 12th week of intrauterine gestation and on, a continuous remodeling of this prototypic structure takes place. A few parts of the primitive biliary structures dilate and slightly roam toward the center of the portal field. These structures are called "peripheral tubular or ductular structures." These biliary structures are the immature form of the interlobular bile ducts. Subsequently, one or two immature structures, mostly peripherally located ductular structures transmute into mature interlobular bile ducts. In the meantime, most of these peripherally located structures will gradually disappear, and an essential contribution to this process is due to the apoptosis, which was initially hypothesized by Professor Valeer Desmet (Leuven, Belgium) as early as 1985 [11–16]. Subsequently, Meckel syndrome, a genetic syndrome with autosomal recessive inheritance, occipital encephalocele, postaxial polydactyly, diffuse cystic renal dysplasia, and malformation of the orthologue development of the ductal plate of the liver, was targeted by my research group in the late years of last century [17]. The malformed ductal plates in the fetal livers with Meckel syndrome showed a marked decrease in the apoptotic rate and Fas expression, a pro-apoptotic marker, and an increase in proliferative activity and expression of Bcl-2, which has an antiapoptotic significance [18]. The conversion of the ductal plate into mature and bile draining interlobular bile ducts is conveyed by the appearance of specific intermediate filaments of the cytoskeleton or keratins or cytokeratins (CKs) [19, 20]. The epithelial cells that are forming the interlobular bile ducts start expressing K-7 and K-19 in addition to K-8 and K-18. The keratins K-8 and K-18 are positive in normal hepatocytes of the adult. Quantification of structures of the biliary system and their maturity may be beneficial in the assessment of the maturation of the intrahepatic biliary tree in neonatal and infantile cholangiopathies, and the lack of an interlobular bile duct is the most worrisome prognosticator in a cholangiopathy independently from the specific etiology or

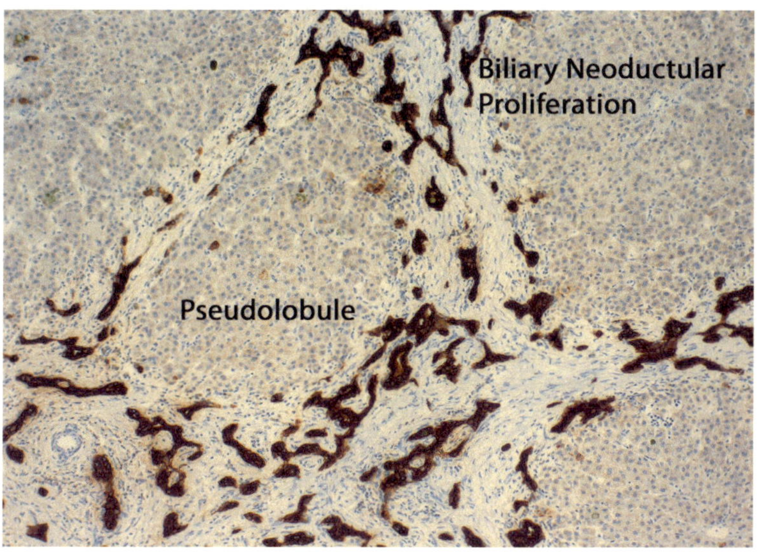

Figure 2.
Keratin 7-immunostaining of the biliary proliferating neoductules (Anti-cytokeratin 7 immunostaining, Avidin-Biotin-Complex, x100 original magnification).

labeling of the disease [21]. **Figure 2** shows the immunohistochemical staining of the biliary proliferation using an antibody against cytokeratin 7.

3. Liver biopsy

Currently, the liver biopsy remains the gold standard for determining the diagnosis of surgical conditions with neonatal cholestasis, such as BA, which is the most critical surgically correctable form of persistent conjugated hyperbilirubinemia. There is an incredible rate of accuracy that comes with the experience of the pathologist and liver biopsy is precise in probably more than 9 cases out of 10, in most tertiary centers of pediatric healthcare, provided that the liver tissue encompasses at least six portal tracts. The experience of the pathologist may be crucial to address the patient to a pediatric surgeon or genetic counseling for neonatal cholestatic liver diseases. The challenge may be quite high that some argued that there might be a continuum with a single underlying cause. According to our previously published data [21], patterns of ductular reactions may muddle the pathologist, and ductal plate remnants, often seen in the liver histology, may indeed recapitulate the embryonic anlage. As a pediatrician and pathologist, the urgency of critical reports is well understood [22]. Medical and surgical causes of neonatal cholestasis need to be ruled out promptly. The central differential diagnoses of BA that need to be kept in mind are: Alagille syndrome, alpha-1-antitrypsin deficiency, cystic fibrosis, sclerosing cholangitis with neonatal onset, and more rarely progressive familial intrahepatic cholestasis (PFIC) types I-III. The differential diagnosis may be complicated and ancillary studies may need mass spectroscopy or other sophisticated techniques.

4. Genetics

As indicated early, BA is usually not hereditary, but some cases and families with recurrence rate have been observed [23]. Four genetic loci are considered as predisposition loci in BA, although no etiologic mutation was identified. The rare occurrence of BA in well-known genetic syndromes seems to suggest coincidental finding, but epigenetic aspects might play a major role in contributing to the increase of BA rate. Chromosomal alterations reported in patients with BA include duplication, deletion, and single copy number variation. Duplications include trisomy 18, trisomy or tetrasomy 22, trisomy 21, trisomy 10q and trisomy 11q23. In trisomy 18, BA has been associated in individuals with congenital heart disease and facial dysmorphism. In trisomy or tetrasomy 22, cat eye syndrome occurs. Facial dysmorphism, congenital heart disease, and cleft palate occurred in trisomy 11q23, while coarctation of the aorta, anal anteposition, and mental retardation have been recorded in patients harboring trisomy 10q. Patients with trisomy 21 syndrome (Down syndrome) showed accompanying atresia of the duodenum and esophagus as well as a heterotaxic setting, which is a condition in which the internal organs are abnormally arranged in the abdomen and chest. Deletion of chromosomal portions has been identified on 18p, 2q73.3, 18q21, 17q12, 1p36, and 20p11.21. Facial dysmorphism, mental retardation, hypothyroidism, and polysplenia were founds in deletion of the 2q37.2, while hyperechogenic kidney and pancreatic hypoplasia were found in the deletion of 17q12. Facial dysmorphism and classic Pitt-Hopkins syndrome were found in the deletion of 1p36 and 18q21, respectively. Laterality defects and panhypopituitarism were findings in the setting of deletion of 20p11.21. Pitt-Hopkins syndrome is a condition characterized by developmental delay and intellectual disability with individuals with breathing problems, recurrent seizures, and distinctive facial features [24–27]. There is a delay in the development of mental and motor skills with numerous affected individuals having features of autistic spectrum disorders. Copy number variations (CNVs) are defined as a type of structural variation: specifically, i.e., a type of duplication or deletion event that affects a considerable number of base pairs. CNVs are a phenomenon in which sections of the genome are repeated, and the number of repeats in the genome varies between individuals in the human population with a specific neurological disorder as seen in Huntington's disease. In this disease, CAG (i.e., cytosine-adenine-guanine) repeats of less than 26 have no effect, but between 27 and 35 there is a risk for the offspring, 36–29 CAG repeats may (or may not) be affected by the disease but harbors 50% of risk to offspring, while 40 or more has a consequence with full penetrance of the disease and a risk of 50% to offspring. CMVs have been identified in a cohort of patients with BA with 29 specific CNVs involving the *JAG1* gene and immunity-related genes. Genome-wide association studies performed in patients affected with BA identified four loci, of which one is in the Han population and three in Caucasians. In the Han ethnics of China, noncoding single nucleotide polymorphisms (SNPs) have been localized to *ADD3* and *XPNPEP1* genes. Noncoding SNPs and a heterozygous deletion have been localized in *ARF6*, *EFEMP1*, and *GPC1* genes, respectively [28–30]. There have been some case reports of BA associated with identified mutation or diagnosed syndrome. The gene *SERPINA1* was considered an aggravating factor for BA, and *JAG1* was questioned in a few patients [31–34]. A compound heterozygous (one copy each of two different alleles) mutation was also questioned in case of *PKHD1* gene [35]. A heterozygous mutation of the gene *MYO5B* was found in a patient suffering from microvillus inclusion disease and progressive familial cholestasis [34]. The Dubin-Johnson syndrome was also found in a patient with BA implying the gene *ABCC2* [34]. Progressive familial cholestasis without microvillus inclusion disease was found in a patient with BA as well. The gene involved *ABCB11* harbored a heterozygous mutation. Heterozygous and hemizygous mutations of the genes *CFC1* and *ZIC3* were found in patients with laterality defects [36, 37]. To be hemizygous for a gene means to have only one copy of one allele of that gene. The Fumarase gene was seen in a patient having a homozygous mutation [38]. The gene *GATA3* was involved as a heterozygous mutation in a patient with HDR syndrome (hypoparathyroidism, sensorineural deafness and renal abnormalities) [39], while the gene *FGFR3* was involved in a patient with achondroplasia [40]. The Mitchell-Riley syndrome was found in an individual with BA and a homozygous mutation of the gene *RFX6* [41]. Fanconi anemia and BA with a biallelic mutation on *ERCC4* were also found [42]. Kartagener syndrome and BA also occurred in the literature [43]. The Zimmermann-Laband syndrome was present in an individual with BA and a heterozygous mutation of *KCNH1* [44]. Kabuki syndrome and BA also occurred in the literature [45, 46]. The Mowat-Wilson syndrome was found in a patient with BA and a heterozygous deletion in the *ZEB2* gene. Two more genes were also seen having a heterozygous mutation in patients with BA including *UGT1A1* and *MLL2* [34]. Finally, three multiple congenital anomaly syndromes have been reported with BA, including Mutchinick syndrome, Goldenhar syndrome, and caudal regression syndrome. Although the presentation of case reports and small case series may indicate a genetic background suggesting that a genetic element plays a significant role in the pathogenesis of BA, we need to argue that the genetics is probably only one of the multiple factors that may occur coincidentally or sequentially. The few reported familial cases of BA have been supportive [46–50] although conflicting sets of monozygotic twins have also been identified [51–53]. Another important aspect is the variations in the incidence of BA among different ethnics and the incidence of HLA B12 and, of course, haplotypes A9-B5 and A28-B35 were also found to be higher in infants with BA compared to a control group [54]. The high incidence rates of BA in some areas of Southeast Asia, as well as Polynesia, are evocative of an inherited predisposition, although a local eating style or viral factor cannot be rules out [51].

The original dichotomic description of BA in embryonic and fetal type or syndromic and non-syndromic forms is still valid [47]. The reader may need to keep in mind that most probably the term "atresia" is a misnomer and a necroinflammatory process of obliterative nature is different from an atretic process in origin from the embryologic point of view. In consideration of the period in which "atresia" occurs, it may be classified as embryonic or fetal and perinatal. In approximately 20% of patients with BA, the embryonic form is responsible, while the rest is due to fetal form, which is also called perinatal form. In the early form, the extrahepatic biliary tree might have undergone abnormal morphogenetic processes. BA patients suffering from this form of BA have associated non-hepatic structural anomalies, of which the most common multiple congenital anomalies is the polysplenia syndrome, which is found in 8–12% of patients with BA. This syndrome is characterized by polysplenia/asplenia associated with cardiac defects (dextrocardia, tetralogy of Fallot, anomalies of the pulmonary vasculature, atrio-/ventricular septal defects) a midline liver, preduodenal portal vein, interruption of the inferior vena cava, and *situs viscerum inversus*, and intestinal malrotation. Other congenital malformations can be detected, such as cardiac anomalies, annular pancreas, immotile cilia syndrome (pointing to Kartagener syndrome), duodenal atresia (leading to trisomy 21 syndrome), esophageal atresia, polycystic kidney disease, cleft palate, and jejunal atresia. The fetal or perinatal form is characterized by patency of the extrahepatic and intrahepatic biliary system at birth, but an inflammatory and sclerosing reaction, caused by perinatal injury, results in the obstruction of the biliary tree. The fetal or perinatal form accounts for four out five cases of BA, and it is not typically associated with congenital anomalies [48, 49].

If about 10% of patients with BA have multiple congenital anomalies, it has been argued that the laterality defects have a phenotype like that detected in the ciliopathies, which is a heterogeneous group of disorders caused by structural and functional abnormalities in genes that encode cilia proteins [23, 50–55]. Embryologically, cilia are evolutionarily conserved. The cilia support in founding the left-right axis in vertebrates and are present on numerous cell types. The cilia are also present in the apical surface of biliary cells or cholangiocytes. In these cells, cilium function is integral to bile flow, bile ductular maturation, and neoductular formation [49]. The *PKHD1* gene is responsible for the autosomal recessive polycystic kidney disease (ARPKD). The expression of the *PKHD1* is polycystin, which was found reduced in the livers of infants with BA with and without associated renal cysts by comparing with liver resections of patients without BA [25, 46]. Studies involving rhesus rotavirus murine models of BA have found the extensive loss of primary cilia from extrahepatic cholangiocytes, which was verified by the finding of decreased ciliation in extrahepatic biliary ducts in infants with BA of perinatal type, although cilia appeared normal in neighboring peribiliary glands [50].

There is quite an overwhelming evidence against a Mendelian paradigm of inheritance of BA. The argument against a Mendelian inheritance is supported by the lack of familial penetrance, despite rare cases of familial BA [52, 53], and discordant presentation of BA among twins, including monozygotic twins [54–57]. On the other side, a growing principle of developmental diseases exhibits unusual patterns of inheritance, including Bardet-Biedl syndrome. The Bardet-Biedl syndrome is a ciliopathy, which is clinically heterogeneous and specifically marked by oligogenic inheritance. The mutations in multiple genes cooperate to generate the phenotype of Bardet-Biedl syndrome. It has been suggested that a similar singularity related to gene-gene interactions, or epistasis, may account for the diversity of presentations in BA [23]. Non-Mendelian inheritance is also detected in Alagille syndrome, which is the

result of a haploid insufficiency of *JAG1* (alternatively its receptor NOTCH2). There is a inconstant intrafamilial clinical presentation [58, 59].
Microchimerism is clearly defined as the occurrence of two genetically different cell populations in the same person. There are a few etiologies, in which it can arise and include blood transfusion, organ transplantation and the bidirectional transfer of cells between mother and fetus during pregnancy as well as the twin-to-twin transfer in utero [56]. Microchimerism has been suggested to explain the phenotypic heterogeneity and nonclassical genetic inheritance of BA [60, 61].

Recently, genome-wide association studies (GWASs) have been milestones in identifying some genes and pathways of several diseases. A GWAS is an observational study of a genome-wide set of genetic variants in diverse individuals to understand if any modification is associated with a trait. Generally, GWASs emphasize the associations between single-nucleotide polymorphisms (SNPs) and traits like major human diseases but can equally be useful for any other genetic variants and any other organisms. SNPs are DNA sequence variations occurring probably 1 in every 100, 200–300 bases along the 3-billion-base human genomic sequence and at least 1% of the population. SNPs make up about 90% of DNA sequence variation as indicated by the Human Genome Project (http://www.ornl.gov, http://linkage.rockefeller.edu/soft/). On the other side, if one of the possible sequences is present in less than 1% of the population (99.9% of people have a C, and 0.1% have a G), then the variation is called a mutation [57, 58].

The Han Chinese population is particularly susceptible to GWAS because of the large size of individuals and homogeneity of this population. A recent study using a GWAS found a potential susceptibility locus for BA between the genes ADD3 and XPNPEP1 located with the chromosomal localization of 10q25.1 with replication in independent Chinese and Thai specimens and identification of BA in a Zebrafish model [59–61]. Interestingly, sequencing of a Han Chinese sample identified that a 5-SNP risk haplotype to be associated with BA and the genotype correlated with reduced levels of *ADD3* expression [61]. The study was attempted to be replicated in a Caucasian cohort [60]. The authors found a stronger signal in the first intron of *ADD3*, although the exact genotype at this SNP was not predictive of the degree of *ADD3* expression. The gene under intense investigation is *ADD3* or adducin 3. Adducins are heteromeric proteins constituted of different subunits (alpha, beta, and gamma). The three subunits are involved in the assembly of the spectrin-actin network in red blood cells and at sites of cell-cell contact in epithelial tissues. Adducins alpha and gamma are universally expressed, while adducin beta is found in the brain and hematopoietic tissues. Adducin 3 is a cytoskeleton-associated protein that endorses the assemblage of the spectrin-actin network. Adducin 3 plays a role in actin filament capping and binds to calmodulin [62–63]. In **Figure 3**, the interaction of adducin 3 with other markers is depicted. This representation is the product of the interaction of several molecules, including ADD1, ADD2, ANKRD29, C1orf85, DDX10, MSANTD1, PSIP1, XPNPEP1, and XP07 [64]. Apart of adducin 1 and 2 that belong to the same family of adducins (heteromeric cytoskeletal proteins), the other genes/proteins are extremely intriguing to study in BA patients and may give us hints to understand the pathogenesis of this challenging cholangiopathy [65]. *ANKRD29* (Ankyrin Repeat Domain 29) is a protein-coding gene with the gene located on chromosome 18q11.2. C1orf85 is a glycosylated lysosomal membrane protein with gene ontology annotations including DNA binding transcription factor activity and, of course, ligand-dependent nuclear receptor transcription coactivator activity. DDX10 is a DEAD box protein, characterized by the conserved motif Asp-Glu-Ala-Asp (DEAD). This class of proteins are putative RNA helicases and are implicated in many cellular processes involving alteration of RNA secondary structure (e.g., translation initiation, nuclear and mitochondrial splicing,

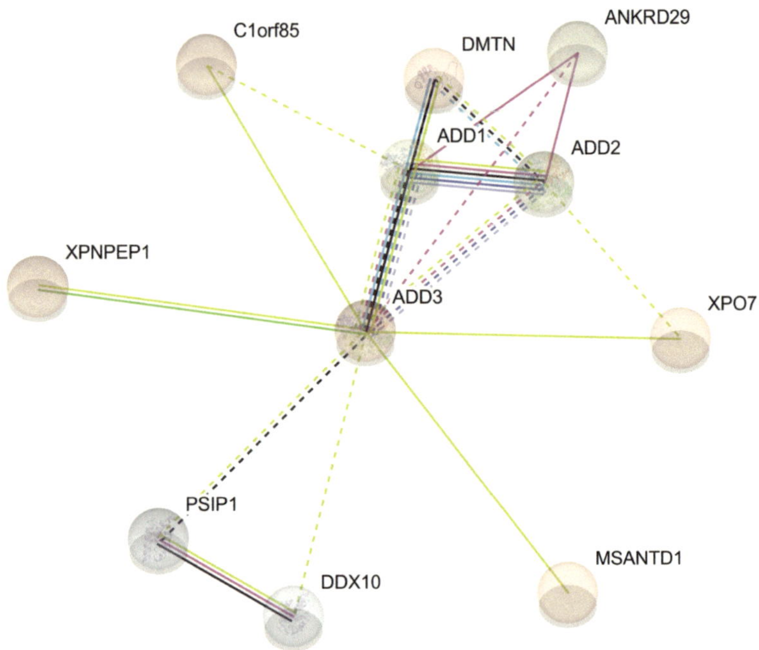

Figure 3.
Interactome of the ADD3 protein with splice isoforms or post-translational modifications are collapsed, while each node represents all the proteins produced by a single, protein-coding gene locus. The edges represent protein-protein interactions with different color according to the interaction type. A red line indicates the presence of fusion evidence, green line a neighborhood evidence, blue line a cooccurrence evidence, purple line an experimental evidence, yellow line a textmining evidence, light blue line a database evidence, and black line a coexpression evidence (see text for details).

and ribosome and spliceosome assembly). In consideration of the distribution patterns, some members of this family are held to be involved in embryogenesis. They may play a role in spermatogenesis, and, overall, cellular growth and division. *MSANTD1* is Myb/SANT DNA Binding Domain Containing 1 and is a protein-coding gene, which is also known as chromosome 4 open reading frame 44. PSIP1 is PC4 and SFRS1 Interacting Protein 1, which is a protein-coding gene. PSIP1 is a transcriptional coactivator involved in the differentiation and neurogenesis of neuroepithelial stem cells and specifically in gene regulation and stress responses of lens epithelial cells. The shielding role during stress-induced apoptosis may raise the suspicion that this pattern may be particularly relevant to investigate in the future. Diseases associated with PSIP1 include atopic dermatitis. PSIP1 also seems interesting because two related pathways with PSIP1 are ERK Signaling and Akt Signaling. XPNPEP1 is a protein coded from a gene *XPNPEP1*. The *XPNPEP1* gene encodes the form in cytosol of a metalloaminopeptidase that catalyzes the cleavage of the N-terminal amino acid adjacent to a proline residue. It seems that this gene product plays a role in the degradation and maturation of tachykinins, neuropeptides, and peptide hormones. There are multiple transcript variants linked to alternative splicing. Finally, XPO7 or Exportin 7 is coded by the *XPO7* gene. The protein has binding and nuclear export signal receptor activity. It serves for the transport of protein and large RNAs through the nuclear pore complexes in an energy-dependent and regulated process. XPO7 mediates the nuclear export of proteins (cargos), which have broad substrate specificity. In the nucleus, this protein binds cooperatively to its cargo and the GTPase Ran in its active GTP-bound form. After curbing of this trimeric complex to the nuclear pore complex through binding to nucleoporins, EXPO7 translocated into the cytoplasm, and the disassembling of the complex and hydrolysis of Ran-GTP to Ran-GDP determines the release of the cargo from the export receptor. Following this action, XPO7 shows an iterative procedure returning to the nuclear compartment and mediate another round of transport.

The GWAS was also able to identify an additional putative gene, which is called glypican 1 (*GPC1*). *GPC1* is located on chromosome 2q37.3 and has been replicated in an independent cohort of patients demonstrating heterozygous deletion of this gene as the sole gene in this region [62]. Glypicans are heparan sulfate proteoglycans. Glypicans are bound to the external surface of the plasmatic membrane of a cell by a glycosylphosphatidylinositol (GPI) linkage [62, 63, 66]. Homologs of glypican molecules have been identified throughout the Eumetazoa, although clear glypican homologs are not definitely found outside the Metazoa. The family of these proteoglycans includes six members (GPC1–GPC6). Glypican family members are tangled in numerous signaling and developmental pathways in hepatocytes and cholangiocytes, and there is role of GPC-3 for being a marker and a therapeutic target of hepatocellular carcinoma [66], In 2018, Sangkhathat et al. used a whole exome sequencing approach to look for other cholestasis entities in 20 cases diagnosed with BA in Thailand. These authors targeted well 19 genes associated with infantile cholestasis syndromes. Variant selection focused on those with allele frequencies in dbSNP150 database of less than 0.01. A polymerase chain reaction (PCR)-direct sequencing was used to verify all selected variants. Of the 20 cases studied, 13 rare variants were detected in nine genes: four in *JAG1* (Alagille syndrome), two in *MYO5B* (progressive familial intrahepatic cholestasis [PFIC] type 6), and one each in *ABCB11* (PFIC type 2), *ABCC2* (Dubin-Johnson syndrome), *ERCC4* (Fanconi anemia), *KCNH1* (Zimmermann-Laband syndrome), *MLL2* (Kabuki syndrome), *RFX6* (Mitchell-Riley syndrome), and *UG1A1* (Crigler-Najjar syndrome). The authors concluded that severe inflammatory cholangiopathy in BA might be a shared pathology among several infantile cholestatic syndromes [34]. Although these results may be controversially discussed, there is time to verify these conclusions. However, far to be univocal the genetic research on BA showed that other genes involved in biliary tract dysmorphogenesis and cholestasis, the immunologic response, vasculogenesis, and left-right patterning might contribute to this disease with worrisome complications and prognosis. Currently, clinical investigations and nonhuman model systems are focusing on *CFC1*, *CFTR*, *JAG1*, *IFN-γ*, *INV*, *MIF*, *VEGF*, *SOX17*, and *ZIC3* [34–40, 65, 67]. Currently, the finalization of genomic studies has not been reached, but the application of GWAS points incontrovertibly toward two candidate genes that may underlie the development of BA in these patients, including *ADD3* and *GPC1*. It may be important to cross the ethnics and investigate other populations. The use of next-generation sequencing (NGS) has been a throughput in technology in the last decade and will have enormous value in BA research. NGS technologies are miniaturized and parallelized sequencing platforms are targeting from 1 million to 43 billion short reads (50–400 bases each) per instrument run. The massive parallel sequencing is carried out via spatially separated, clonally amplified DNA templates or single DNA molecules localized in a flow cell. NGS is different from the PCR-based Sanger sequencing that is based on polyacrylamide gel electrophoretic separation of chain-termination products available in individual sequencing reactions. NGS strengths include the possibility to detect abnormalities across the entire genome, including substitutions, deletions, insertions, duplications, copy number changes (gene and exon), and chromosome inversions/translocations using less DNA than required for traditional DNA sequencing approaches (e.g., Sanger sequencing). NGS gives data on some molecular aberrations with no currently clinical significance. It requires sophisticated bioinformatics systems, fast data processing, and large data storage capabilities, which can be costly without adequate bioinformatics support. Despite drawbacks, NGS has been used extensively in research and diagnostics [68–72].

5. Epigenetics and genetic modifiers of biliary atresia

Epigenetic modification (e.g., methylation) may be at the basis of some BA patients [73]. Epigenetics is the investigation of inherited variations in the expression of genes that do not involve deviations to the underlying DNA sequence. It means that there is a change in phenotype without evidence of a deviation in genotype. Epigenetics specifically affects how cells translate the genes. There is a natural occurrence of epigenetics, but several factors including age, lifestyle, environment, and disease state influence the epigenetic flow in an organism. Epigenetic changes can affect how cells terminally differentiate or how cancer can occur. There are at least three systems including DNA methylation, modification of histones, and non-coding RNA (ncRNA)-associated gene silencing that are considered to initiate and endure epigenetic change. Epigenetic studies in BA may be particularly challenging because hepatocyte or cholangiocyte DNA of patients may be needed. It has been hypothesized that some genes that are relevant for the biliary function may be involved. These genes may be *A1AT*, *JAG1*, and *CFTR*, but also targeting the bile canaliculus transporters [50, 74–77].

6. Non-genetic contributive factors of biliary atresia

It would be incomplete this chapter, if BA would not be discussed exploring the non-genetic causes of this condition. Although poorly understood, some non-genetic factors may contribute to the development of this surgically correctable neonatal biliary disease. There are several categories, including viruses, toxins, immunological dysregulations, and feto-maternal factors [1, 78–82]. Cytomegalovirus (CMV) is a genus of viruses in the order *Herpesvirales*, in the family *Herpesviridae*, in the subfamily *Betaherpesvirinae*. Both monkeys and humans serve as natural hosts and eight species in this genus are known. Among them, there is the human cytomegalovirus, which is the species that infects humans. CMV has been implicated in BA a few instances in the literature [83–91]. Challenges are the inconsistency of its detection in clinical samples or routine liver biopsy. Other viruses include rotavirus and reovirus, but also other viruses, such as hepatotropic viruses, have been questioned as etiologic factors for this obstructive cholangiopathy of the neonatal age [83, 92–103]. Another etiologic consideration are toxins. Bush tea or other components containing pyrrolizidine alkaloids, deriving mostly from the *Senecio* species, *Crotalaria* species, *Heliotropium lasiocarpum*, or *Symphytum* (comfrey), are a known source to hepatologists and toxicologists [104]. Hepatotoxic pyrrolizidine alkaloids have been found in 150 species of plants. BA may be considered in analogy to the obliterative process seen in pyrrolizidine alkaloids or similar plants [105]. In Australia, toxins present in plants of the *Dysphania* species have been associated with a damage of the biliary system in animals, but the significance for humans is still uncertain [106, 107]. The incidence of viral infection is not epidemic, and BA does not occur outside of the perinatal period. Thus, a virologic etiology may not be widely supported by a strong evidence. An immune-related or an autoimmunologic disorder is also still plausible due to the absence of recurrence after transplantation [50]. In some infants from Egypt, the cause of BA has been demonstrated to be result of aflatoxin-induced cholangiopathy acquired prenatally in infants who harbor glutathione S-transferase M1 deficiency [108].

7. Final remarks and future perspectives

BA remains a very challenging disease not only from the clinical point of views but also for the pathological one and transcriptome analysis cannot provide a univocal answer [109]. The importance to differentiate surgically correctable cholangiopathies in the neonatal age is crucial for the prognosis of these patients. The introduction of the Kasai HPE has revolutionized the outcome of patients harboring this condition. The timing when the Kasai HPE is performed has been emphasized as critical. Alternatively, liver transplantation is the only hope for liver cirrhosis developed on the ground of a BA. The underlying cause(s) and outcome contributor(s) to BA remain poorly understood, but new technologies are on the front to target this field. Two genes that we currently consider of significant interest for BA are *ADD3* gene and *GPC1* gene. The feasibility of animal models may also be extremely used in studying the cohorts of animals that may develop this condition in prospective multigeneration investigations. The use of in-depth learning methodologies will be vital in analyzing the massive mole of data that can come out from these experiments, but the use of highly sophisticated computational platforms is opening the horizon for this disease.

Acknowledgements

This work is dedicated to the career of Prof. Dr. J. Hager (**Figure 4**), formerly Director of the Department of Pediatric and Youth Surgery, of the University of Innsbruck, Austria. Prof. Hager was born in 1946 and his career has been fulfilled of enormous and vivid achievements as well as honors, such as the European pediatric surgery diploma, Theodor-Billroth Prize of the Austrian Society for Surgery, and the Spitzy Prize. He has more than 150 peer-reviewed publications with countless lectures and presentations. His mentoring and teaching activity resulted in numerous fellows, who came out from his school in Innsbruck.

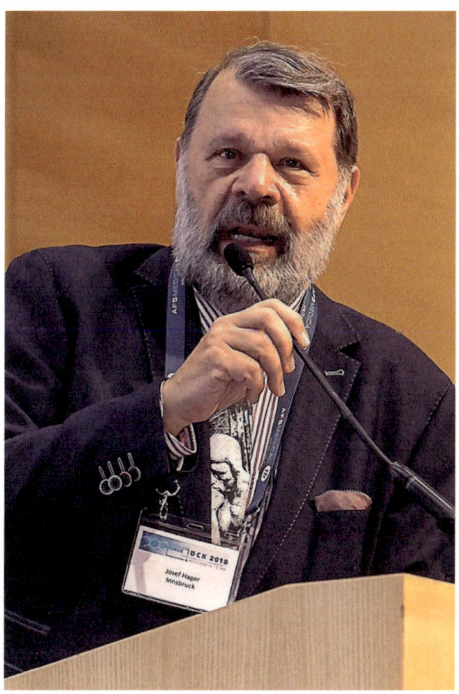

Figure 4.
Professor Dr. med. Josef Hager during a presentation.

Author details

Consolato M. Sergi

1 Department of Laboratory Medicine and Pathology, University of Alberta, Edmonton, Canada

2 Stollery Children's Hospital, Edmonton, Alberta, Canada

*Address all correspondence to: sergi@ualberta.ca

References

[1] Chardot C. Biliary atresia. Orphanet Journal of Rare Diseases. 2006;**1**:28. DOI: 10.1186/1750-1172-1-28

[2] Carvalho NMN, Torres SM, Cavalcante JCB, Ximenes ACM, Landim Junior JA, Moreira S. Hepatoportoenterostomy surgery technique. Journal of Pediatric Surgery. 2018;**10**. DOI: 10.1016/j.jpedsurg.2018.10.041

[3] Omar H, Siglin S, Laurie T, Kavin H. 26-year-old survivor of Kasai procedure with native liver. ACG Case Reports Journal. 2016;**3**(3):221-223. DOI: 10.14309/crj.2016.56

[4] Garcia AV, Cowles RA, Kato T, Hardy MA. Morio Kasai: A remarkable impact beyond the Kasai procedure. Journal of Pediatric Surgery. 2012;**47**(5):1023-1027. DOI: 10.1016/j.jpedsurg.2012.01.065

[5] Sergi C, Adam S, Kahl P, Otto HF. The remodeling of the primitive human biliary system. Early Human Development. 2000;**58**(3):167-178. Available from: https://www.ncbi.nlm.nih.gov/pubmed/10936437

[6] Hammar JA. Uber die erste Entstehung der nicht kapillaren intrahepatischen Gallengange beim Menschen. Zeitschrift für Mikroskopisch-Anatomische Forschung. 1926;**5**:59-89

[7] Nakanuma Y, Hoso M, Sanzen T, Sasaki M. Microstructure and development of the normal and pathologic biliary tract in humans, including blood supply. Microscopy Research and Technique. 1997;**38**(6):552-570. DOI: 10.1002/(SICI)1097-0029(19970915)38:6<552::AID-JEMT2>3.0.CO;2-H

[8] Desmet VJ, van Eyken P, Roskams T. Histopathology of vanishing bile duct diseases. Advances in Clinical Pathology. 1998;**2**(2):87-99. Available from: https://www.ncbi.nlm.nih.gov/pubmed/10358336

[9] Dorn L, Menezes LF, Mikuz G, Otto HF, Onuchic LF, Sergi C. Immunohistochemical detection of polyductin and co-localization with liver progenitor cell markers during normal and abnormal development of the intrahepatic biliary system and in adult hepatobiliary carcinomas. Journal of Cellular and Molecular Medicine. 2009;**13**(7):1279-1290. DOI: 10.1111/j.1582-4934.2008.00519.x

[10] Johnson CA, Gissen P, Sergi C. Molecular pathology and genetics of congenital hepatorenal fibrocystic syndromes. Journal of Medical Genetics. 2003;**40**(5):311-319. Available from: https://www.ncbi.nlm.nih.gov/pubmed/12746391

[11] Faber W, Sharafi S, Stockmann M, Dennecke T, Bahra M, Klein F, et al. Patient age and extent of liver resection influence outcome of liver resection for hepatocellular carcinoma in non-cirrhotic liver. Hepato-Gastroenterology. 2014;**61**(135):1925-1930. Available from: http://www.ncbi.nlm.nih.gov/pubmed/25713889

[12] Desmet VJ. Ludwig symposium on biliary disorders—Part I. Pathogenesis of ductal plate abnormalities. Mayo Clinic Proceedings. 1998;**73**(1):80-89. Available from: https://www.ncbi.nlm.nih.gov/pubmed/9443684

[13] Desmet VJ. Histopathology of cholestasis. Verhandlungen der Deutschen Gesellschaft für Pathologie. 1995;**79**:233-240. Available from: https://www.ncbi.nlm.nih.gov/pubmed/8600686

[14] Desmet VJ. What is congenital hepatic fibrosis? Histopathology. 1992;**20**(6):465-477. Available from:

https://www.ncbi.nlm.nih.gov/pubmed/1607148

[15] Desmet VJ. Congenital diseases of intrahepatic bile ducts: Variations on the theme "ductal plate malformation". Hepatology. 1992;**16**(4):1069-1083. Available from: https://www.ncbi.nlm.nih.gov/pubmed/1398487

[16] Desmet VJ. Intrahepatic bile ducts under the lens. Journal of Hepatology. 1985;**1**(5):545-559. Available from: https://www.ncbi.nlm.nih.gov/pubmed/4056355

[17] Sergi C, Adam S, Kahl P, Otto HF. Study of the malformation of ductal plate of the liver in Meckel syndrome and review of other syndromes presenting with this anomaly. Pediatric and Developmental Pathology. 2000;**3**(6):568-583. Available from: https://www.ncbi.nlm.nih.gov/pubmed/11000335

[18] Sergi C, Kahl P, Otto HF. Contribution of apoptosis and apoptosis-related proteins to the malformation of the primitive intrahepatic biliary system in Meckel syndrome. The American Journal of Pathology. 2000;**156**(5):1589-1598. DOI: 10.1016/S0002-9440(10)65031-6

[19] Van Eyken P, Sciot R, Callea F, Van der Steen K, Moerman P, Desmet VJ. The development of the intrahepatic bile ducts in man: A keratin-immunohistochemical study. Hepatology. 1988;**8**(6):1586-1595. Available from: https://www.ncbi.nlm.nih.gov/pubmed/2461337

[20] Van Eyken P, Sciot R, Desmet V. Intrahepatic bile duct development in the rat: A cytokeratin-immunohistochemical study. Laboratory Investigation. 1988;**59**(1): 52-59. Available from: https://www.ncbi.nlm.nih.gov/pubmed/2455831

[21] Sergi C, Benstz J, Feist D, Nutzenadel W, Otto HF, Hofmann WJ. Bile duct to portal space ratio and ductal plate remnants in liver disease of infants aged less than 1 year. Pathology. 2008;**40**(3):260-267. DOI: 10.1080/00313020801911538

[22] Sergi C. Promptly reporting of critical laboratory values in pediatrics: A work in progress. World Journal of Clinical Pediatrics. 2018;**7**(5):105-110. DOI: 10.5409/wjcp.v7.i5.105

[23] Girard M, Panasyuk G. Genetics in biliary atresia. Current Opinion in Gastroenterology. 2018. DOI: 10.1097/MOG.0000000000000509

[24] Schonewolf-Greulich B, Bisgaard AM, Moller RS, Duno M, Brondum-Nielsen K, Kaur S, et al. Clinician's guide to genes associated with rett-like phenotypes—Investigation of a Danish cohort and review of the literature. Clinical Genetics. 2019;**95**(2):221-230. DOI: 10.1111/cge.13153

[25] Kasem E, Kurihara T, Tabuchi K. Neurexins and neuropsychiatric disorders. Neuroscience Research. 2018;**127**:53-60. DOI: 10.1016/j.neures.2017.10.012

[26] Dean L. Pitt-Hopkins syndrome. In: Pratt V, McLeod H, Rubinstein W, Dean L, Kattman B, Malheiro A, editors. Medical Genetics Summaries. National Center for Biotechnology Information (USA). Bethesda, MD; 2012. Available from: https://www.ncbi.nlm.nih.gov/pubmed/28520343

[27] Sweetser DA, Elsharkawi I, Yonker L, Steeves M, Parkin K, Thibert R. Pitt-Hopkins syndrome. In: Adam MP, Ardinger HH, Pagon RA, Wallace SE, Bean LJH, Stephens K, et al., editors. GeneReviews®. Seattle, WA, USA: University of Washington; 1993. Available from: https://www.ncbi.nlm.nih.gov/pubmed/22934316

[28] Ningappa M, So J, Glessner J, Ashokkumar C, Ranganathan S, Min J,

et al. The role of ARF6 in biliary atresia. PLoS ONE. 2015;**10**(9):e0138381. DOI: 10.1371/journal.pone.0138381

[29] Chen Y, Gilbert MA, Grochowski CM, McEldrew D, Llewellyn J, Waisbourd-Zinman O, et al. A genome-wide association study identifies a susceptibility locus for biliary atresia on 2p16.1 within the gene EFEMP1. PLoS Genetics. 2018;**14**(8):e1007532. DOI: 10.1371/journal.pgen.1007532

[30] Ke J, Zeng S, Mao J, Wang J, Lou J, Li J, et al. Common genetic variants of GPC1 gene reduce risk of biliary atresia in a Chinese population. Journal of Pediatric Surgery. 2016;**51**(10):1661-1664. DOI: 10.1016/j.jpedsurg.2016.05.009

[31] Campbell KM, Arya G, Ryckman FC, Alonso M, Tiao G, Balistreri WF, et al. High prevalence of alpha-1-antitrypsin heterozygosity in children with chronic liver disease. Journal of Pediatric Gastroenterology and Nutrition. 2007;**44**(1):99-103. DOI: 10.1097/01.mpg.0000243434.54958.21

[32] Kohsaka T, Yuan ZR, Guo SX, Tagawa M, Nakamura A, Nakano M, et al. The significance of human jagged 1 mutations detected in severe cases of extrahepatic biliary atresia. Hepatology. 2002;**36**(4 Pt 1):904-912. DOI: 10.1053/jhep.2002.35820

[33] Dedic T, Jirsa M, Keil R, Rygl M, Snajdauf J, Kotalova R. Alagille syndrome mimicking biliary atresia in early infancy. PLoS ONE. 2015;**10**(11):e0143939. DOI: 10.1371/journal.pone.0143939

[34] Sangkhathat S, Laochareonsuk W, Maneechay W, Kayasut K, Chiengkriwate P. Variants associated with infantile cholestatic syndromes detected in extrahepatic biliary atresia by whole exome studies: A 20-case series from Thailand. Journal of Pediatric Genetics. 2018;7(2):67-73. DOI: 10.1055/s-0038-1632395

[35] Hartley JL, O'Callaghan C, Rossetti S, Consugar M, Ward CJ, Kelly DA, et al. Investigation of primary cilia in the pathogenesis of biliary atresia. Journal of Pediatric Gastroenterology and Nutrition. 2011;**52**(4):485-488. DOI: 10.1097/MPG.0b013e318200eb6f

[36] Davit-Spraul A, Baussan C, Hermeziu B, Bernard O, Jacquemin E. CFC1 gene involvement in biliary atresia with polysplenia syndrome. Journal of Pediatric Gastroenterology and Nutrition. 2008;**46**(1):111-112. DOI: 10.1097/01.mpg.0000304465.60788.f4

[37] Ware SM, Peng J, Zhu L, Fernbach S, Colicos S, Casey B, et al. Identification and functional analysis of ZIC3 mutations in heterotaxy and related congenital heart defects. American Journal of Human Genetics. 2004;**74**(1):93-105. DOI: 10.1086/380998

[38] Vara R, Grammatikopoulos T, Gallagher C, Agalou S, Zen Y, Davenport M, et al. Fumarase deficiency associated with noninflammatory biliary atresia. Journal of Pediatric Gastroenterology and Nutrition. 2014;**58**(3):e32-e34. DOI: 10.1097/MPG.0b013e31826f7526

[39] Higuchi Y, Hasegawa K, Yamashita M, Fujii Y, Tanaka H, Tsukahara H. HDR syndrome in a Japanese girl with biliary atresia: A case report. BMC Pediatrics. 2016;**16**:14. DOI: 10.1186/s12887-016-0550-9

[40] Kylat RI. Achondroplasia and biliary atresia: A rare association and review of literature. Journal of Pediatric Genetics. 2017;**6**(2):122-125. DOI: 10.1055/s-0036-1597930

[41] Khan N, Dandan W, Al Hassani N, Hadi S. A newly-discovered mutation in the RFX6 gene of the rare Mitchell-Riley syndrome. Journal of Clinical Research in Pediatric Endocrinology. 2016;**8**(2):246-249. DOI: 10.4274/jcrpe.2387

[42] Bogliolo M, Schuster B, Stoepker C, Derkunt B, Su Y, Raams A, et al. Mutations in ERCC4, encoding the DNA-repair endonuclease XPF, cause Fanconi anemia. American Journal of Human Genetics. 2013;**92**(5):800-806. DOI: 10.1016/j.ajhg.2013.04.002

[43] Gershoni-Baruch R, Gottfried E, Pery M, Sahin A, Etzioni A. Immotile cilia syndrome including polysplenia, situs inversus, and extrahepatic biliary atresia. American Journal of Medical Genetics. 1989;**33**(3):390-393. DOI: 10.1002/ajmg.1320330320

[44] Balasubramanian M, Parker MJ. Zimmermann-Laband syndrome in a child previously described with brachydactyly, extrahepatic biliary atresia, patent ductus arteriosus and seizures. Clinical Dysmorphology. 2010;**19**(1):48-50. DOI: 10.1097/MCD.0b013e328333c239

[45] Selicorni A, Colombo C, Bonato S, Milani D, Giunta AM, Bedeschi MF. Biliary atresia and Kabuki syndrome: Another case with long-term follow-up. American Journal of Medical Genetics. 2001;**100**(3):251. Available from: https://www.ncbi.nlm.nih.gov/pubmed/11343312

[46] McGaughran JM, Donnai D, Clayton-Smith J. Biliary atresia in Kabuki syndrome. American Journal of Medical Genetics. 2000;**91**(2):157-158. Available from: https://www.ncbi.nlm.nih.gov/pubmed/10748418

[47] Howard ER. Biliary atresia. In: Stringer MD, Oldham KT, Mouriquand PDE, Howard ER, editors. Pediatric Surgery and Urology: Long Term Outcomes. London, UK: WB Saunders; 1998. pp. 402-416

[48] Carvalho E, Santos JL, Silveira TR, Kieling CO, Silva LR, Porta G, et al. Biliary atresia: The Brazilian experience. Jornal de Pediatria. 2010;**86**(6):473-479. DOI: 10.2223/JPED.2054

[49] de Carvalho E, Ivantes CA, Bezerra JA. Extrahepatic biliary atresia: Current concepts and future directions. Jornal de Pediatria. 2007;**83**(2):105-120. DOI: 10.2223/JPED.1608

[50] Mezina A, Karpen SJ. Genetic contributors and modifiers of biliary atresia. Digestive Diseases. 2015;**33**(3):408-414. DOI: 10.1159/000371694

[51] Tsai EA, Grochowski CM, Falsey AM, Rajagopalan R, Wendel D, Devoto M, et al. Heterozygous deletion of FOXA2 segregates with disease in a family with heterotaxy, panhypopituitarism, and biliary atresia. Human Mutation. 2015;**36**(6):631-637. DOI: 10.1002/humu.22786

[52] Schwarz KB, Haber BH, Rosenthal P, Mack CL, Moore J, Bove K, et al. Extrahepatic anomalies in infants with biliary atresia: Results of a large prospective North American multicenter study. Hepatology. 2013;**58**(5):1724-1731. DOI: 10.1002/hep.26512

[53] Chu AS, Russo PA, Wells RG. Cholangiocyte cilia are abnormal in syndromic and non-syndromic biliary atresia. Modern Pathology. 2012;**25**(5):751-757. DOI: 10.1038/modpathol.2011.212

[54] Tumgor G, Cogulu O, Onay H, Ekmekci AY, Aydogdu S, Durmaz B, et al. Unusual presentation of biliary atresia splenic malformation syndrome with autosomal dominant hypospadias. Genetic Counseling. 2011;**22**(4):347-351. Available from: https://www.ncbi.nlm.nih.gov/pubmed/22303794

[55] Stoll C, Morali A, Leheup B, Lucron H. Extrahepatic biliary atresia with laterality sequence anomalies. Genetic Counseling. 2001;**12**(2):157-161. Available from: https://www.ncbi.nlm.nih.gov/pubmed/11491311

[56] Knippen MA. Microchimerism: Sharing genes in illness and in health. ISRN Nursing. 2011;**2011**:893819. DOI: 10.5402/2011/893819

[57] Corfield A, Meyer P, Kassam S, Mikuz G, Sergi C. SNPs: At the origins of the databases of an innovative biotechnology tool. Frontiers in Bioscience (Scholar Edition). 2010;**2**:1-4. Available from: https://www.ncbi.nlm.nih.gov/pubmed/20036923

[58] Meyer P, Sergi C, Garbe C. Polymorphisms of the BRAF gene predispose males to malignant melanoma. Journal of Carcinogenesis. 2003;**2**(1):7. DOI: 10.1186/1477-3163-2-7

[59] Tang V, Cofer ZC, Cui S, Sapp V, Loomes KM, Matthews RP. Loss of a candidate biliary atresia susceptibility gene, add3a, causes biliary developmental defects in Zebrafish. Journal of Pediatric Gastroenterology and Nutrition. 2016;**63**(5):524-530. DOI: 10.1097/MPG.0000000000001375

[60] Tsai EA, Grochowski CM, Loomes KM, Bessho K, Hakonarson H, Bezerra JA, et al. Replication of a GWAS signal in a Caucasian population implicates ADD3 in susceptibility to biliary atresia. Human Genetics. 2014;**133**(2):235-243. DOI: 10.1007/s00439-013-1368-2

[61] Cheng G, Tang CS, Wong EH, Cheng WW, So MT, Miao X, et al. Common genetic variants regulating ADD3 gene expression alter biliary atresia risk. Journal of Hepatology. 2013;**59**(6):1285-1291. DOI: 10.1016/j.jhep.2013.07.021

[62] Dwivedi PP, Grose RH, Filmus J, Hii CS, Xian CJ, Anderson PJ, et al. Regulation of bone morphogenetic protein signalling and cranial osteogenesis by Gpc1 and Gpc3. Bone. 2013;**55**(2): 367-376. DOI: 10.1016/j.bone.2013.04.013

[63] Filmus J, Capurro M, Rast J. Glypicans. Genome Biology. 2008;**9**(5):224. DOI: 10.1186/gb-2008-9-5-224

[64] Szklarczyk D, Franceschini A, Wyder S, Forslund K, Heller D, Huerta-Cepas J, et al. STRING v10: Protein-protein interaction networks, integrated over the tree of life. Nucleic Acids Research. 2015;**43**(Database issue):D447-D452. DOI: 10.1093/nar/gku1003

[65] Mack CL, Anderson KM, Aubrey MT, Rosenthal P, Sokol RJ, Freed BM. Lack of HLA predominance and HLA shared epitopes in biliary atresia. Springerplus. 2013;**2**(1):42. DOI: 10.1186/2193-1801-2-42

[66] Filmus J, Capurro M. Glypican-3: A marker and a therapeutic target in hepatocellular carcinoma. The FEBS Journal. 2013;**280**(10):2471-2476. DOI: 10.1111/febs.12126

[67] Bergmann C. Genetics of autosomal recessive polycystic kidney disease and its differential diagnoses. Frontiers in Pediatrics. 2017;**5**:221. DOI: 10.3389/fped.2017.00221

[68] Celesti F, Celesti A, Wan J, Villari M. Why deep learning is changing the way to approach NGS data processing: A review. IEEE Reviews in Biomedical Engineering. 2018;**11**:68-76. DOI: 10.1109/RBME.2018.2825987

[69] Fernandez-Marmiesse A, Gouveia S, Couce ML. NGS technologies as a turning point in rare disease research, diagnosis and treatment. Current Medicinal Chemistry. 2018;**25**(3): 404-432. DOI: 10.2174/09298673246661 70718101946

[70] Sanchez-Mazas A, Nunes JM. Does NGS typing highlight our understanding of HLA population diversity?: Some good reasons to say yes and a few to say be careful. Human Immunology. 2018. DOI: 10.1016/j.humimm.2018.10.004

[71] Santani A, Simen BB, Briggs M, Lebo M, Merker JD, Nikiforova M, et al. Designing and implementing NGS tests for inherited disorders—A practical framework with step-by-step guidance for clinical laboratories. The Journal of Molecular Diagnostics. 2018;**10**. DOI: 10.1016/j.jmoldx.2018.11.004

[72] Morganti S, Tarantino P, Ferraro E, D'Amico P, Viale G, Trapani D, et al. Complexity of genome sequencing and reporting: Next generation sequencing (NGS) technologies and implementation of precision medicine in real life. Critical Reviews in Oncology/Hematology. 2019;**133**:171-182. DOI: 10.1016/j.critrevonc.2018.11.008

[73] Yang Y, Shen F, Huang W, Qin S, Huang JT, Sergi C, et al. Glucose is involved in the dynamic regulation of m6A in patients with type 2 diabetes. The Journal of Clinical Endocrinology and Metabolism. 2018;**10**. DOI: 10.1210/jc.2018-00619

[74] Rock N, McLin V. Liver involvement in children with ciliopathies. Clinics and Research in Hepatology and Gastroenterology. 2014;**38**(4):407-414. DOI: 10.1016/j.clinre.2014.04.001

[75] Cui S, Leyva-Vega M, Tsai EA, Eau Claire SF, Glessner JT, Hakonarson H, et al. Evidence from human and zebrafish that GPC1 is a biliary atresia susceptibility gene. Gastroenterology. 2013;**144**(5):1107e3-1115e3. DOI: 10.1053/j.gastro.2013.01.022

[76] Zhao D, Long XD, Xia Q. Recent advances in etiology of biliary atresia. Clinical Pediatrics (Phila). 2015;**54**(8):723-731. DOI: 10.1177/0009922814548841

[77] Miethke AG, Huppert SS. Fishing for biliary atresia susceptibility genes. Gastroenterology. 2013;**144**(5):878-881. DOI: 10.1053/j.gastro.2013.03.017

[78] Petersen C, Davenport M. Aetiology of biliary atresia: What is actually known? Orphanet Journal of Rare Diseases. 2013;**8**:128. DOI: 10.1186/1750-1172-8-128

[79] Petersen C. Biliary atresia: The animal models. Seminars in Pediatric Surgery. 2012;**21**(3):185-191. DOI: 10.1053/j.sempedsurg.2012.05.002

[80] Bezerra JA, Wells RG, Mack CL, Karpen SJ, Hoofnagle JH, Doo E, et al. Biliary atresia: Clinical and research challenges for the 21(st) century. Hepatology. 2018;**10**. DOI: 10.1002/hep.29905

[81] Mack CL, Sokol RJ. Unraveling the pathogenesis and etiology of biliary atresia. Pediatric Research. 2005;**57**(5 Pt 2):87R-94R. DOI: 10.1203/01.PDR.0000159569.57354.47

[82] Nakamura K, Tanoue A. Etiology of biliary atresia as a developmental anomaly: Recent advances. Journal of Hepato-Biliary-Pancreatic Sciences. 2013;**20**(5):459-464. DOI: 10.1007/s00534-013-0604-4

[83] Averbukh LD, Wu GY. Evidence for viral induction of biliary atresia: A review. Journal of Clinical and Translational Hepatology. 2018;**6**(4):410-419. DOI: 10.14218/JCTH.2018.00046

[84] Goel A, Chaudhari S, Sutar J, Bhonde G, Bhatnagar S, Patel V, et al. Detection of cytomegalovirus in liver tissue by polymerase chain reaction in infants with neonatal cholestasis. The Pediatric Infectious Disease Journal. 2018;**37**(7):632-636. DOI: 10.1097/INF.0000000000001889

[85] Lakshminarayanan B, Davenport M. Biliary atresia: A comprehensive review. Journal of Autoimmunity. 2016;**73**:1-9. DOI: 10.1016/j.jaut.2016.06.005

[86] Zani A, Quaglia A, Hadzic N, Zuckerman M, Davenport M.

Cytomegalovirus-associated biliary atresia: An aetiological and prognostic subgroup. Journal of Pediatric Surgery. 2015;**50**(10):1739-1745. DOI: 10.1016/j.jpedsurg.2015.03.001

[87] Moore SW, Zabiegaj-Zwick C, Nel E. Problems related to CMV infection and biliary atresia. South African Medical Journal. 2012;**102**(11 Pt 2): 890-892. DOI: 10.7196/samj.6163

[88] De Tommaso AM, Andrade PD, Costa SC, Escanhoela CA, Hessel G. High frequency of human cytomegalovirus DNA in the liver of infants with extrahepatic neonatal cholestasis. BMC Infectious Diseases. 2005;**5**:108. DOI: 10.1186/1471-2334-5-108

[89] Amer OT, Abd El-Rahma HA, Sherief LM, Hussein HF, Zeid AF, Abd El-Aziz AM. Role of some viral infections in neonatal cholestasis. The Egyptian Journal of Immunology. 2004;**11**(2):149-155. Available from: https://www.ncbi.nlm.nih.gov/pubmed/16734127

[90] Oliveira NL, Kanawaty FR, Costa SC, Hessel G. Infection by cytomegalovirus in patients with neonatal cholestasis. Arquivos de Gastroenterologia. 2002;**39**(2):132-136. Available from: https://www.ncbi.nlm.nih.gov/pubmed/12612719

[91] Domiati-Saad R, Dawson DB, Margraf LR, Finegold MJ, Weinberg AG, Rogers BB. Cytomegalovirus and human herpesvirus 6, but not human papillomavirus, are present in neonatal giant cell hepatitis and extrahepatic biliary atresia. Pediatric and Developmental Pathology. 2000;**3**(4): 367-373. Available from: https://www.ncbi.nlm.nih.gov/pubmed/10890252

[92] Saito T, Terui K, Mitsunaga T, Nakata M, Ono S, Mise N, et al. Evidence for viral infection as a causative factor of human biliary atresia. Journal of Pediatric Surgery. 2015;**50**(8):1398-1404. DOI: 10.1016/j.jpedsurg.2015.04.006

[93] Nakashima T, Hayashi T, Tomoeda S, Yoshino M, Mizuno T. Reovirus type-2-triggered autoimmune cholangitis in extrahepatic bile ducts of weanling DBA/1J mice. Pediatric Research. 2014;**75**(1-1):29-37. DOI: 10.1038/pr.2013.170

[94] Rauschenfels S, Krassmann M, Al-Masri AN, Verhagen W, Leonhardt J, Kuebler JF, et al. Incidence of hepatotropic viruses in biliary atresia. European Journal of Pediatrics. 2009;**168**(4):469-476. DOI: 10.1007/s00431-008-0774-2

[95] Saito T, Shinozaki K, Matsunaga T, Ogawa T, Etoh T, Muramatsu T, et al. Lack of evidence for reovirus infection in tissues from patients with biliary atresia and congenital dilatation of the bile duct. Journal of Hepatology. 2004;**40**(2):203-211. Available from: https://www.ncbi.nlm.nih.gov/pubmed/14739089

[96] Szavay PO, Leonhardt J, Czech-Schmidt G, Petersen C. The role of reovirus type 3 infection in an established murine model for biliary atresia. European Journal of Pediatric Surgery. 2002;**12**(4):248-250. DOI: 10.1055/s-2002-34477

[97] Huang YH, Shih HH, Tiao MM, Huang CC, Kuo KC, Huang FC, et al. Toll-like receptor 7 agonist induces hypoplasia of the biliary system in a neonatal mouse model. Journal of Microbiology, Immunology, and Infection. 2018;**51**(2):166-173. DOI: 10.1016/j.jmii.2016.07.002

[98] Danial E, Fleck-Derderian S, Rosenthal P. Has rotavirus vaccination decreased the prevalence of biliary atresia? Journal of Clinical Gastroenterology. 2018;**10**. DOI: 10.1097/MCG.0000000000001121

[99] Clemente MG, Patton JT, Anders RA, Yolken RH, Schwarz KB. Rotavirus infects human biliary epithelial cells and stimulates secretion of cytokines IL-6 and IL-8 via MAPK pathway. BioMed Research International. 2015;**2015**:697238. DOI: 10.1155/2015/697238

[100] Oetzmann von Sochaczewski C, Pintelon I, Brouns I, Dreier A, Klemann C, Timmermans JP, et al. Rotavirus particles in the extrahepatic bile duct in experimental biliary atresia. Journal of Pediatric Surgery. 2014;**49**(4):520-524. DOI: 10.1016/j.jpedsurg.2013.09.064

[101] Mohanty SK, Donnelly B, Bondoc A, Jafri M, Walther A, Coots A, et al. Rotavirus replication in the cholangiocyte mediates the temporal dependence of murine biliary atresia. PLoS ONE. 2013;**8**(7):e69069. DOI: 10.1371/journal.pone.0069069

[102] Hertel PM, Estes MK. Rotavirus and biliary atresia: Can causation be proven? Current Opinion in Gastroenterology. 2012;**28**(1):10-17. DOI: 10.1097/MOG.0b013e32834c7ae4

[103] Allen SR, Jafri M, Donnelly B, McNeal M, Witte D, Bezerra J, et al. Effect of rotavirus strain on the murine model of biliary atresia. Journal of Virology. 2007;**81**(4):1671-1679. DOI: 10.1128/JVI.02094-06

[104] Sergi C, Beedgen B, Linderkamp O, Hofmann WJ. Fatal course of veno-occlusive disease of the liver (endophlebitis hepatica obliterans) in a preterm infant. Pathology, Research and Practice. 1999;**195**(12):847-851. DOI: 10.1016/S0344-0338(99)80108-3

[105] Walesky C, Goessling W. Nature and nurture: Environmental toxins and biliary atresia. Hepatology. 2016;**64**(3):717-719. DOI: 10.1002/hep.28701

[106] Koo KA, Waisbourd-Zinman O, Wells RG, Pack M, Porter JR. Reactivity of biliatresone, a natural biliary toxin, with glutathione, histamine, and amino acids. Chemical Research in Toxicology. 2016;**29**(2):142-149. DOI: 10.1021/acs.chemrestox.5b00308

[107] Harper P, Plant JW, Unger DB. Congenital biliary atresia and jaundice in lambs and calves. Australian Veterinary Journal. 1990;**67**(1):18-22. Available from: https://www.ncbi.nlm.nih.gov/pubmed/2334368

[108] Kotb MA, Kotb A. Extrahepatic biliary atresia is an aflatoxin induced cholangiopathy in infants with null GSTM1 genotype with disrupted P53 and GSTPi to mothers heterozygous for GSTM1 polymorphism: Damage control is mediated through neutrophil elastase and CD14+ activated monocytes: Kotb disease. The Medical journal of Cairo University. 2015;**83**(2):137-145

[109] Carvalho E, Liu C, Shivakumar P, Sabla G, Aronow B, Bezerra JA. Analysis of the biliary transcriptome in experimental biliary atresia. Gastroenterology. 2005;**129**(2):713-717. DOI: 10.1016/j.gastro.2005.05.052

Chapter 3

Nonalcoholic Fatty Liver Disease

Marco Antonio López Hernández

Abstract

The nonalcoholic fatty liver disease (NAFLD) is the liver disorder that is most common in Western countries; has a global prevalence of approximately 25%; and is strongly associated to obesity and metabolic syndrome. According to the Third National Health and Nutrition Examination Survey (NHANES III), the prevalence of NAFLD is more common in obese individuals with a prevalence of 39.4% than in lean individuals with a prevalence of 7.7%. Nonalcoholic fatty liver disease is the hepatic manifestation of the metabolic syndrome and is defined as the accumulation of fat in the liver. The NAFLD is defined by an accumulation of fat in liver with >5% of steatosis by histologic examination or by proton density fat fraction >5.6%. The diagnosis of NAFLD implies the exclusion of secondary causes like alcohol consumption. The NAFLD includes two different pathological conditions with different prognosis: the nonalcoholic fatty liver (NAFL) and the nonalcoholic steatohepatitis (NASH), the last one has a wide spectrum of severity.

Keywords: NAFLD, NAFL, NASH, liver disease, fatty liver disease

1. Introduction

The nonalcoholic fatty liver disease is the most common liver alteration in the Western countries, with an incidence from the 17–46% of the adult patients [1]. Analysis of the Third National Health and Nutrition Examination Survey presented in the 2018 Annual Meeting of the American Association for the Study of Liver Diseases [2] demonstrated nonalcoholic fatty liver disease prevalence of 7.7% among lean individuals vs. 39.4% among obese individuals. The prevalence of NAFLD among lean individuals without any components of metabolic syndrome was 2.2%, and no evidence of increased overall or cardiovascular-related mortality among this subgroup was found. The presence of diabetes mellitus (DM) was identified as independent risk factor for NAFLD in both lean and obese individuals in multivariate logistic regression analysis (**Table 1**).

The nonalcoholic fatty liver disease is defined as the accumulation of fat in the liver and can be considered a hepatic manifestation of the metabolic syndrome. The prevalence of NAFLD is 20–30% in adults and is higher in industrialized countries [3].

The screening for NAFLD in the community has been questioned for high costs of testing, but the progressive form of NAFLD, particularly when associated with advanced fibrosis, should be identified in patients at risk, because of its prognostic implications.

2. Definition of NAFLD

The NAFLD is characterized by an excessive liver fat accumulation and insulin resistance. Liver biopsy is the standard for diagnosis of NALFD, and it is defined by

NAFLD prevalence, %	Lean subjects (n = 3242)		Obese subjects (n = 2592)	
	Male	**Female**	**Male**	**Female**
Total	7.32	7.54	50.48*	35.2
Metabolically normal	4.39	7.12	23.89	15.14
DM + hypertension/hyperlipidemia	15.32	23.65	65.61	49.34
Hypertension + hyperlipidemia, only	12.76*	0.92	32.26	25.7
DM, only	15.01	6.50	5.32	57.96*
Hypertension, only	5.17	1.54	29.76	33.48
Hyperlipidemia, only	7.47	9.28	43.91*	20.75

**P < .05 for difference in men vs. women within lean or obese subsets.*

Table 1.
Prevalence of NAFLD according to features of metabolic syndrome in lean and obese subjects in NANHES III.

NAFL	NASH
Pure steatosis	Early NASH (F0–F1) no or mild fibrosis
Steatosis with mild lobular inflammation	Fibrotic NASH (F2–F3) significant or advanced fibrosis
	NASH cirrhosis (F4)
	Hepatocellular carcinoma

Table 2.
Classification of NAFLD.

the presence of more than 5% of steatosis of the hepatocytes by histologic examination or more than 5.6% assessed by proton magnetic resonance spectroscopy or quantitative fat/water selective magnetic resonance imaging.

The diagnosis of NAFLD implies the differentiation of two different liver disorders associated to the liver fat accumulation: the nonalcoholic fatty liver and the nonalcoholic steatohepatitis. NAFL can be subdivided in pure steatosis and steatosis with mild lobular inflammation. The spectrum of the NASH has includes a wide range of stages from: early NASH: no or mild fibrosis (stages F0-F1), fibrotic NASH; that includes significant (F2) or advanced (F3) fibrosis, NASH-cirrhosis (F4), and hepatocellular carcinoma (**Table 2**).

The NAFLD also called primary NALFD is associated with risk factors and components of metabolic syndrome, like waist circumference >94 cm in men or >80 in women, arterial pressure >130/85 mmHg or treated for hypertension, serum triacylglycerols >150 mg/dL, and HDL cholesterol <40 mg/dL in men or <50 mg/dL in women.

The screening for metabolic syndrome independent of liver enzymes in all the patients with liver steatosis is recommended, and, because the nonalcoholic fatty liver disease is the main reason of unexpected elevated liver enzymes, the patients with persistently high elevation of liver enzymes must be screened. The screening of NAFLD with liver enzymes and USG in the patients with obesity or metabolic syndrome is also recommended.

3. Pathogenesis

The high-calorie diet with an excess of saturated fats and refined carbohydrates has been associated with weight gain and obesity and more recently with NAFLD [4, 5]. The "multiple hit" hypothesis considers multiple insults acting together on

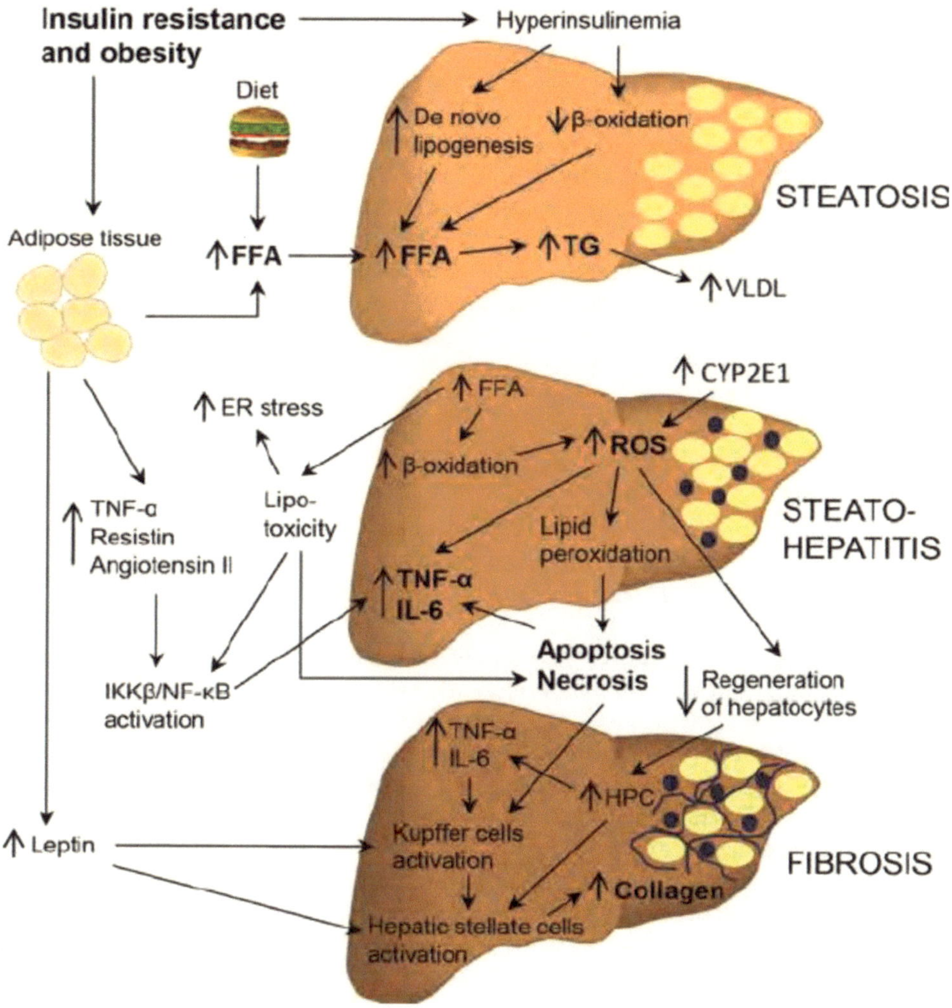

Figure 1.
Multiple hit theory of pathogenesis of NAFLD.

genetically predisposed subjects to induce NAFLD and provide a more accurate explanation of NAFLD pathogenesis [6].

Dietary habits and genetic and environmental factors can lead to insulin resistance, obesity with adipocyte proliferation, and changes in the gut microbiota. The insulin resistance is a key factor in the pathogenesis of NAFLD; the insulin resistance results in a hepatic de novo lipogenesis and impaired inhibition of adipose tissue lipolysis, with consequent increased flux of fatty acids to the liver [7]. Insulin resistance also promotes adipose tissue dysfunction that results in an impaired secretion of adipokines and inflammatory cytokines [8] (**Figure 1**).

Genetic factors and epigenetic changes, in predisposed individuals, affect hepatocyte fat content and contribute to create an inflammatory environment in the liver with possible progression to hepatocellular death mediated for both direct toxicity and apoptosis activating mechanisms, activation of hepatic stellate cells, and deposition of fibrous matrix.

Altered microbiota in the gut leads to the fatty acid accumulation in the small bowel, increased permeability and absorption of fatty acids, and raised circulating levels of molecules which contribute to the activation of inflammatory pathways and release of proinflammatory cytokines [9].

Genetic variants, especially in the form of single nucleotide polymorphisms, influence hepatic fatty acids flux, oxidative stress, response to endotoxins, and cytokine production and activity and are determinants of NAFLD development and progression. Epigenetic modifications are defined as stable changes which do not alter the basic DNA sequences at transcriptional level, such as histone modifications, DNA methylation, and activity of microRNAs, and these changes contribute to a high degree of developmental and environmentally driven plasticity in the cell homeostasis [10, 11].

Genotyping may be considered in selected patients and clinical studies but is not recommended routinely. The carriers of the PNPLA3 I148M and the TM6SF2 E167K genotypes have a higher liver fat content and increased risk of NASH. The NAFLD due to these variants is not systematically associated with features of insulin resistance.

4. Diagnosis

The standard procedure for the diagnosis of NASH is the liver biopsy and is the only procedure that can differentiate the NAFL from NASH, despite limitations due to sampling variability [12].

The histologic NAFL features include steatosis alone, steatosis with lobular or portal inflammation, without ballooning, or steatosis with ballooning but without inflammation.

For evaluation of severity of the disease, the NAFLD Activity Score (NAS) scoring system can be used; this score should not be used for diagnosis. This score is correlated with homeostasis model assessment of insulin resistance (HOMA-IR) and the aminotransferase level [13].

Noninvasive diagnostic procedures must be considered in primary care settings; they identify the risk of NAFLD among individuals with increased metabolic risk; in secondary and tertiary care settings, they identify those with worse prognosis; monitor disease progression; and predict response to therapeutic interventions.

When NAFLD is suspected as the primary disease or as a coexisting condition, steatosis should be documented. The presence of NASFLD also predicts cardiovascular events, arterial hypertension, and diabetes mellitus. The quantification of fat content is not of interest, in clinical practice, except for the evaluation of treatment efficacy, and is therefore not generally recommended. Steatosis of the liver should be documented by ultrasonography, because it is a cheaper and more available method than MRI. US has limited sensitivity and does not reliably detect steatosis when <20% [14, 15].

US is the preferred first-line diagnostic procedure for imaging of NAFLD, as it provides additional diagnostic information. A quantitative estimation of liver fat can only be obtained by 1H-MRS. This technique is of value in clinical trials and experimental studies but is expensive and not recommended in the clinical setting.

The diagnosis of NASH implicates closer follow-up, provides important prognostic information, and indicates an increased risk of fibrosis progression, cirrhosis, and possibly hepatic comorbidities. It may also prompt possibly a greater need for more intensive therapy. Clinical, biochemical, or imaging measures cannot distinguish NASH from steatosis [16, 17].

NASH must be diagnosed by a liver biopsy showing steatosis, hepatocyte ballooning, and lobular inflammation. Biomarkers and scores of fibrosis, as well as transient elastography, are acceptable noninvasive procedures for the identification of cases at low risk of advanced fibrosis/cirrhosis.

5. Metabolic disorders linked to NAFLD

5.1 Obesity

Insulin resistance has been associated with NAFLD, not only in the liver but also in adipose tissues and muscle and also with the metabolic syndrome. The metabolic syndrome is defined as the cluster of any three of the following five features: impaired fasting glucose or type 2 diabetes mellitus, hypertriglyceridemia, low high-density lipoprotein (HDL) cholesterol, increased waist circumference, and high blood pressure [18].

Obesity is the major phenotype and risk condition for NAFLD, driven by insulin resistance, and increases the risk of advanced disease. Most lean persons with NAFLD display insulin resistance and altered body fat distribution even though they have less severe metabolic disturbance than overweight NAFLD.

5.2 Diabetes mellitus

Type 2 diabetes mellitus patients are insulin resistant, often obese, dyslipidemic, display increased liver enzymes, and tend to accumulate hepatic fat, without relation with the body mass index [19–21].

In persons with NAFLD, screening for diabetes is mandatory, and in patients with type 2 diabetes mellitus, the presence of NAFLD should be looked for irrespective of liver enzyme levels, since those patients are at high risk of disease progression.

5.3 Cardiovascular disease

Atherogenic lesions such as increased carotid intima-media thickness, coronary artery and abdominal aortic and aortic valve calcifications, and endothelial dysfunction are more common in NAFLD. The prevalence and incidence of cardiovascular disease is higher in NAFLD than in matched controls and driven by the association between NAFLD and metabolic syndrome components. In most studies, biochemical markers of atherosclerosis or inflammation and increased levels of procoagulant/prothrombotic factors are more common in NAFLD than in persons without steatosis. They are largely independent of traditional risk factors, duration of diabetes, glycemic control, drug treatment, and metabolic syndrome components. The consensus is that cardiovascular disease should be identified in NAFLD regardless of the presence of traditional risk factors. Conversely NAFLD screening should be performed in persons at high CVD risk [22–24].

5.4 Natural history

In general, NAFLD is a slowly progressive disease, but in 20% of cases fibrosis rapidly progresses. The rate of progression corresponds to one fibrosis stage every 14 years in NAFL and every 7 years in NASH and is doubled by arterial hypertension. Compared with the general population, NASH is associated with an increased standardized mortality ratio. US-diagnosed NAFLD is not associated with increased mortality, presumably because progression to NASH and fibrosis is rare for steatosis alone (**Figure 2**) [25–27].

Metabolic reprogramming for adaptation to the local environment has been recognized as a hallmark of cancer. Although alterations in fatty acid metabolism in cancer cells have received less attention compared to other metabolic alterations such as glucose or glutamine metabolism, recent studies have uncovered the importance of lipid metabolic reprogramming in carcinogenesis.

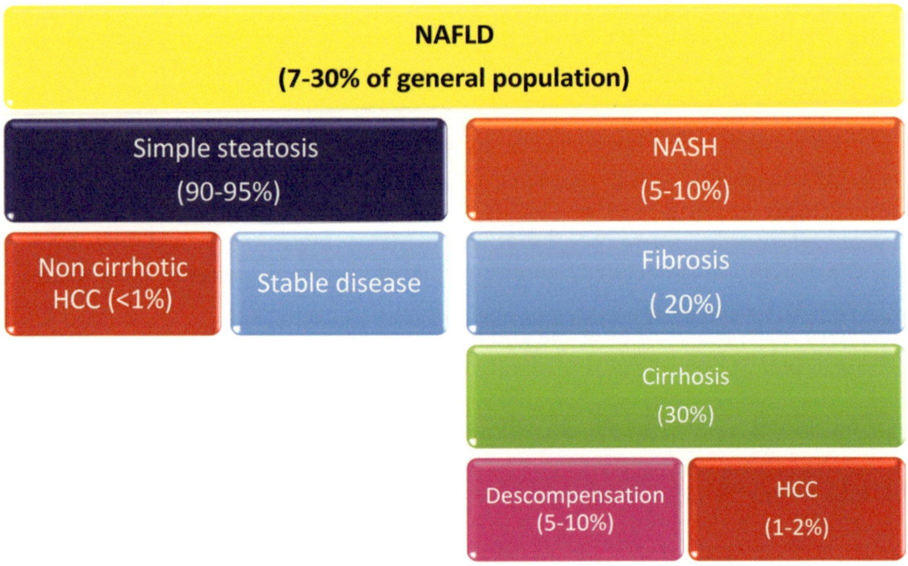

Figure 2.
Natural history of NAFLD. HCC denotes hepatocellular carcinoma.

Obesity and nonalcoholic steatohepatitis (NASH) are well-known risk factors of hepatocellular carcinoma (HCC), and individuals with these conditions exhibit an increased intake of dietary FAs accompanied by enhanced lipolysis of visceral adipose tissue due to insulin resistance, resulting in enormous exogenous fatty acid supplies to hepatocytes via the portal vein and lymph vessels. However, the way in which HCC cells adapt to such a condition and exploit it to aid their progression is not understood. In addition, accumulating evidence supports the importance of lipid metabolic reprogramming in various situations of hepatocarcinogenesis.

5.5 Treatment

Successful treatment of NASH should improve outcomes. The resolution of the histological lesions defining NASH is now accepted as a surrogate end point, particularly in clinical trials. Few well-designed randomized controlled trials are available, with improvement/regression of hepatic necroinflammation and/or fibrosis as primary outcomes.

5.6 Diet and lifestyle changes

Epidemiological evidence suggests a tight relationship between unhealthy lifestyle and NAFLD, which makes lifestyle correction mandatory in all patients. Relatively small amounts of weight loss reduce liver fat and improve hepatic insulin resistance [28].

For the patients with NAFLD, structured programs for lifestyle changes toward healthy diet and habitual physical exercise are recommended. The counseling for healthy diet and physical activity is the election therapy in patients without NASH or fibrosis and with no pharmacotherapy for their liver condition. In overweight or obese NAFLD, weight loss, with a target of 7–10% of the basal weight, is recommended; this results in histology and liver enzyme improvement. Dietary recommendations should consider the caloric restriction and the exclusion of processed food and food and beverages high in added fructose which are NAFLD-promoting components. A macronutrient composition is recommended according to the

Mediterranean diet. Both resistance training and aerobic exercise effectively reduce the amount of fat in the liver. The training must be maintained in the long-term and then is recommended that the choice of training should be tailored based on patients' preferences.

5.7 Drug therapy

Pharmacotherapy should be reserved for patients with NASH, particularly for those with significant fibrosis (stage F2 and higher). Patients with less severe disease, but at high risk of disease progression, could also be candidates to prevent disease progression.

While no firm recommendations can be made, pioglitazone or vitamin E or their combination could be used for NASH.

The optimal duration of therapy is unknown; in patients with increased ALT at baseline, after 6 months of therapy, treatment should be stopped if there is no reduction in aminotransferases; no recommendations can be made in patients with normal ALT at baseline.

The statins have not been showed benefit in liver harm in patients with NAFLD, but may be confidently used to reduce LD cholesterol and prevent cardiovascular risk. There is not data to support the use of n-3 polyunsaturated fatty acids specifically for NASH, but reduce both liver and plasma lipids [29].

By improving obesity and diabetes, bariatric surgery reduces liver fat and is likely to reduce NASH progression; prospective data have shown an improvement in all histological lesions of NASH, including fibrosis [29].

5.8 Drugs in study

In the 2018 Annual Meeting of the American Association for the Study of Liver Diseases, phase II data in therapies with drugs for NAFLD and NASH were presented (**Table 3**).

5.9 Farnesoid X receptor agonists

Farnesoid X receptors (FXRs) are nuclear hormone receptors expressed in high amounts in body tissues that participate in bilirubin metabolism including the liver,

Agent	MOA	N	Study population
GS-9674	FXR agonist	140	NASH
Obeticholic acid	FXR agonist	84	NASH, fibrosis
Tropifexor	FXR agonist	198	NASH
NGM282	FGF19 analogue	38, 85	NASH
MGL-3196	THR-β agonist	125	NASH, hepatic fat fraction ≥10%
VK2809	THR-β agonist	35	NAFLD, liver fat >8%, elevated LDL-C and TG
GS-0976	ACC inhibitor	75	NASH, no cirrhosis
Aramchol	SCD1 inhibitor	247	NASH, overweight or obesity, prediabetes or diabetes
Semaglutide	GLP-1 receptor agonist	957	Obesity, no diabetes

Table 3.
Phase II Data on Investigational NAFLD/NASH Therapies Presented at AASLD 2018.

intestines, and kidneys. Bile acids are the natural ligands of the FXRs. XRs play a critical role in carbohydrate and lipid metabolism and regulation of insulin sensitivity. FXRs also modulate live growth and regeneration during liver injury.

The farnesoid X receptor agonist GSK-9674 was compared with placebo at doses of 30 and 100 mg and showed ≥30% relative reduction in liver fat, and markers of fibrosis also improved [30].

Obeticholic acid (OCA) is a semisynthetic bile acid analogue which has the chemical structure 6α-ethyl-chenodeoxycholic acid. The natural bile acid, chenodeoxycholic acid, was identified in 1999 as the most active physiological ligand for the farnesoid X receptor, which is involved in many physiological and pathological processes. In a double-blind, placebo-controlled, phase II study, the OCA was compared with placebo; at week 16, patients with vs. without cirrhosis (F4 vs. F1–F3) showed no trend for differences in ALT, bilirubin, platelets, and INR [31].

The FLIGHT study on tropifexor (TXR), a three-part randomized, placebo-controlled, double-blind, dose-ranging phase IIb study in adults with NASH, weighing 40–150 kg with liver fat ≥10%, showed reduction in liver fat, ALT, and GGT compared with placebo [32].

5.10 Fibroblast growth factor (FGF) analogues

NGM282 is a non-tumorigenic analogue of human FGF19 demonstrating significant reductions in hepatic steatosis, liver transaminases, and fibrosis markers after 12 weeks of treatment at doses of 3 and 6 mg. The use of NGM282 for 12 weeks at doses of 1 and 3 mg showed clinically meaningful improvements in fibrosis in NASH patients and in all components of the NASH, and this was preceded by rapid and significant improvements in liver transaminases and imaging-based parameters [33].

5.11 Tyroid hormone receptor beta (THR-β)

In a randomized, multicenter, placebo-controlled phase IIa study, at Week 12 a higher proportion of patients with liver fat >30% compared with placebo is shown [34].

MGL-3196 is a liver-directed, orally active, highly selective THR-β agonist which may reduce lipotoxicity in NASH by increasing hepatic fat metabolism. At Week 36, MGL-3196 treatment compared with placebo resulted in significant and sustained reductions in hepatic fat on MRI-PDFF, liver enzymes, fibrosis biomarkers, atherogenic lipids, and improvement in NASH on liver biopsy. In the patients treated with MGL-3193 was observed ≥30% fat reduction (MRI-PDFF) at Week 12 and improved NASH histologic response at Week 36 were predicted [35].

5.12 Acetyl-CoA carboxylase (ACC) inhibitor

Elevated plasma levels of medium- and long-chain acylcarnitines are markers of impaired mitochondrial beta oxidation of fatty acids. GS-0976 inhibits cytoplasmic ACC1 and mitochondrial ACC2 thereby reducing fatty acid synthesis and augmenting beta oxidation, respectively. NASH patients who responded to GS-0976 demonstrated a reduction in plasma acylcarnitine species with reduction of liver fat by MRI-PDFF also. This effect is consistent with an improvement in the efficiency of mitochondrial beta oxidation. The reductions in plasma acylcarnitine species provide further evidence to support, in patients with NASH for the therapeutic targeting of ACC1 and ACC2 [36].

5.13 Stearoyl-coenzyme A desaturase 1 (SCD-1) modulator

Aramchol (arachidyl amido cholanoic acid) is a novel fatty acid bile acid conjugate, inducing beneficial modulation of intrahepatic lipid metabolism. The ARREST study enrolled 247 NASH patients who were overweight/obese and had prediabetes or diabetes with HbA1C at baseline of 6.6%. More than 50% were hypertensive and had dyslipidemia. Baseline histology demonstrated a population with advanced disease, with 60% having stage 2 and 3 fibrosis and 70% having NAS $\geq$ 5.

The study ARREST, is a randomized, global phase IIb study with aramchol in patients with NASH and diabetes or prediabetes, compared aramchol at doses of 400 and 600 mg versus placebo, in the aramchol patients the proportion with >5% of reduction in liver fat by MRI, the resolution of NASH than in the placebo group [37].

5.14 Glucagon-like peptide type 1 (GLP-1) receptor agonist

The glucagon-like peptide 1 analogues semaglutide and liraglutide improve glycemic control and reduce elevated liver enzymes in subjects with type 2 diabetes and reduce body weight in subjects with or without diabetes. Semaglutide at doses of 0.2–0.4 mg daily reduced ALT in subjects with obesity and high ALT to an extent that was broadly comparable across weight loss categories and resulted after 52 weeks in dose-related ALT normalization in up to 46% of subjects. These data suggest a potential role for semaglutide in the treatment of NAFLD with elevated liver enzymes [38].

5.15 Bariatric surgery

Medical therapy, including the newly available drugs, has only limited effects and does neither influence survival or the development of complications or the progression of NASH to liver cirrhosis or the development of hepatocellular carcinomas in NASH. Importantly, even existing diabetic complications such as nephropathy as well as the features of NASH can be reversed by metabolic surgery.

Metabolic surgery is a very effective treatment for NAFLD in general, but in particular for NASH, the beneficial and significant changes in steatosis and NAS after metabolic surgery have been shown with steatosis decreased from 60 to 10% after surgical treatment, and the NASH diminished from 5 to 1, essentially normalizing the liver histology in patients with NASH. Metabolic surgery has even shown to reduce liver fibrosis. A meta-analysis also demonstrated this effect: each of the 16 studies included demonstrated a diminution of steatosis after metabolic surgery [39, 40].

6. Conclusions

The nonalcoholic fatty liver disease is the liver disorder most common in Western countries, has a global prevalence of approximately 25%, and is strongly associated to obesity and metabolic syndrome. Successful treatment of NASH should improve outcomes. Lifestyle changes are the foundation of any treatment plan and weight loss $\geq$3–10% associated with histologic improvement in NAFLD. In the guides of the European Association for Study of Liver disease (EASLD) and the American Association for the Study of Liver Disease (AASLD) is cited recommendations for the use of vitamin E (NASH without diabetes), pioglitazone (NASH with or without diabetes), and bariatric surgery.

Author details

Marco Antonio López Hernández
Internal Medicine Division, Ecatepec General Hospital, Mexico

*Address all correspondence to: niklaus2003@yahoo.com.mx

References

[1] Vernon G, Baranova A, Younossi ZM. Systematic review: The epidemiology and natural history of non-alcoholic fatty liver disease and non-alcoholic steatohepatitis in adults. Alimentary Pharmacology & Therapeutics. 2011;**34**:274-285

[2] Golabi P, Paik J, Rashmi R, et al. Prevalence and long-term outcomes of non-alcoholic fatty liver disease (NAFLD) among lean individuals without any components of metabolic syndrome. In: Program and Abstracts of the 2018 Annual Meeting of the American Association for the Study of Liver Diseases; November 9-13, 2018; San Francisco, California. Abstract 0179

[3] Angulo P. Nonalcoholic fatty liver disease. The New England Journal of Medicine. 2002;**346**:1221-1231

[4] Barrera F, George J. The role of diet and nutritional intervention for the management of patients with NAFLD. Clinics in Liver Disease. 2014;**18**:91-112

[5] Chiu S, Sievenpiper JL, de Souza RJ, Cozma AI, Mirrahimi A, Carleton AJ, et al. Effect of fructose on markers of non-alcoholic fatty liver disease (NAFLD): A systematic review and meta-analysis of controlled feeding trials. European Journal of Clinical Nutrition. 2014;**68**:416-423

[6] Buzzetti E, Pinzani M, Tsochatzis EA. The multiple-hit pathogenesis of non-alcoholic fatty liver disease (NAFLD). Metabolism. 2016;**65**(8):1038-1048

[7] Bugianesi E, Moscatiello S, Ciaravella MF, et al. Insulin resistance in nonalcoholic fatty liver disease. Current Pharmaceutical Design. 2010;**16**:1941-1951

[8] Guilherme A, Virbasius JV, Puri V, et al. Adipocyte dysfunctions linking obesity to insulin resistance and type 2 diabetes. Nature Reviews. Molecular Cell Biology. 2008;**9**:367-377

[9] Kirpich IA, Marsano LS, McClain CJ. Gut-liver axis, nutrition, and non-alcoholic fatty liver disease. Clinical Biochemistry. 2015;**48**(13-14):923-930

[10] Anstee QM, Daly AK, Day CP. Genetics of alcoholic and nonalcoholic fatty liver disease. Seminars in Liver Disease. 2011;**31**:128-146

[11] Zeybel M, Mann DA, Mann J. Epigenetic modifications as new targets for liver disease therapies. Journal of Hepatology. 2013;**59**:1349-1353

[12] Ratziu V, Charlotte F, Heurtier A, Gombert S, Giral P, Bruckert E, et al. Sampling variability of liver biopsy in nonalcoholic fatty liver disease. Gastroenterology. 2005;**28**:1898-1906

[13] Brunt EM, Kleiner DE, Wilson LA, Belt P, Neuschwander-Tetri BA, Network NCR. Nonalcoholic fatty liver disease (NAFLD) activity score and the histopathologic diagnosis in NAFLD: Distinct clinicopathologic meanings. Hepatology. 2011;**53**:810-820

[14] Saadeh S, Younossi ZM, Remer EM, Gramlich T, Ong JP, Hurley M, et al. The utility of radiological imaging in nonalcoholic fatty liver disease. Gastroenterology. 2002;**123**:745-750

[15] Fishbein M, Castro F, Cheruku S, Jain S, Webb B, Gleason T, et al. Hepatic MRI for fat quantitation: Its relationship to fat morphology, diagnosis, and ultrasound. Journal of Clinical Gastroenterology. 2005;**39**:619-625

[16] Machado MV, Cortez-Pinto H. Non-invasive diagnosis of non-alcoholic fatty liver disease. A critical appraisal. Journal of Hepatology. 2013;**58**:1007-1019

[17] European Association for the Study of the Liver, Asociacion Latinoamericana para el Estudio del Higado. EASL-ALEH Clinical Practice Guidelines: Non-invasive tests for evaluation of liver disease severity and prognosis. Journal of Hepatology. 2015;**63**:237-264

[18] Gaggini M, Morelli M, Buzzigoli E, DeFronzo RA, Bugianesi E, Gastaldelli A. Non-alcoholic fatty liver disease (NAFLD) and its connection with insulin resistance, dyslipidemia, atherosclerosis and coronary heart disease. Nutrients. 2013;**5**:1544-1560

[19] Ghouri N, Preiss D, Sattar N. Liver enzymes, nonalcoholic fatty liver disease, and incident cardiovascular disease: A narrative review and clinical perspective of prospective data. Hepatology. 2010;**52**:1156-1161

[20] Gastaldelli A, Cusi K, Pettiti M, Hardies J, Miyazaki Y, Berria R, et al. Relationship between hepatic/visceral fat and hepatic insulin resistance in nondiabetic and type 2 diabetic subjects. Gastroenterology. 2007;**133**:496-506

[21] Kotronen A, Juurinen L, Hakkarainen A, Westerbacka J, Corner A, Bergholm R, et al. Liver fat is increased in type 2 diabetic patients and underestimated by serum alanine aminotransferase compared with equally obese nondiabetic subjects. Diabetes Care. 2008;**31**:165-169

[22] Oni ET, Agatston AS, Blaha MJ, Fialkow J, Cury R, Sposito A, et al. A systematic review: Burden and severity of subclinical cardiovascular disease among those with nonalcoholic fatty liver; should we care? Atherosclerosis. 2013;**230**:258-267

[23] Targher G, Day CP, Bonora E. Risk of cardiovascular disease in patients with nonalcoholic fatty liver disease. The New England Journal of Medicine. 2010;**363**:1341-1350

[24] Bhatia LS, Curzen NP, Calder PC, Byrne CD. Non-alcoholic fatty liver disease: A new and important cardiovascular risk factor? European Heart Journal. 2012;**33**:1190-1200

[25] Singh S, Allen AM, Wang Z, Prokop LJ, Murad MH, Loomba R. Fibrosis progression in nonalcoholic fatty liver vs nonalcoholic steatohepatitis: A systematic review and meta-analysis of paired-biopsy studies. Clinical Gastroenterology and Hepatology. 2015;**13**:643-654, e641–e649; quiz e639–e640

[26] Haflidadottir S, Jonasson JG, Norland H, Einarsdottir SO, Kleiner DE, Lund SH, et al. Long-term follow-up and liver-related death rate in patients with non-alcoholic and alcoholic related fatty liver disease. BMC Gastroenterology. 2014;**14**:166

[27] Kim D, Kim WR, Kim HJ, Therneau TM. Association between noninvasive fibrosis markers and mortality among adults with nonalcoholic fatty liver disease in the United States. Hepatology. 2013;**57**:1357-1313

[28] Petersen KF, Dufour S, Befroy D, Lehrke M, Hendler RE, Shulman GI. Reversal of nonalcoholic hepatic steatosis, hepatic insulin resistance, and hyperglycemia by moderate weight reduction in patients with type 2 diabetes. Diabetes. 2005;**54**:603-608

[29] Marchesini G, Day CP, Dufour JF et al. EASL–EASD–EASO Clinical Practice Guidelines for the management of non-alcoholic fatty liver disease. Journal of Hepatology. 2016;**64**:1388-1402

[30] Patel K, Harrison SA, Trotter JF, et al. The Non-Steroidal FXR Agonist GS-9674 leads to significant reductions in hepatic steatosis, serum bile acids, and liver biochemistry in a Phase 2, randomized, placebo-controlled trial of patients with NASH. In: Program and Abstracts of the 2018 Annual Meeting of the American Association for the Study of Liver Diseases; November 9-13, 2018; San Francisco, California. Abstract 736

[31] Halegoua De Marzio D, Thuluvath PJ, Abdelmalek MF, et al. Obeticholic acid was safe and well tolerated in patients with nonalcoholic steatohepatitis and compensated cirrhosis: A secondary analysis of the control study. In: Program and Abstracts of the 2018 Annual Meeting of the American Association for the Study of Liver Diseases; November 9-13, 2018; San Francisco, California. Abstract 71

[32] Sanyal A, Lopez P, Lawitz E, et al. Tropifexor (TXR), an FXR agonist for the treatment of nash - interim results from first two parts of Phase 2b Study Flight-FXR. In: Program and Abstracts of the 2018 Annual Meeting of the American Association for the Study of Liver Diseases; November 9-13, 2018; San Francisco, California. Abstract LB 23

[33] Harrison FA, Trotter JF, Paredes AH et al. NGM282 Rapidly improves NAFLD activity score (NAS) and fibrosis in 12 weeks in Patients with biopsy-confirmed nonalcoholic steatohepatitis (NASH): Results of a Phase 2 Multi-Center Dose Finding Study. In: Program and Abstracts of the 2018 Annual Meeting of the American Association for the Study of Liver Diseases; November 9-13, 2018; San Francisco, California. Abstract 104

[34] Loomba R, Neutel J, Bernard D, et al. K2809, a novel liver-directed thyroid receptor beta agonist, significantly reduces liver fat in patients with non-alcoholic fatty liver disease: A phase 2 Randomized, Placebo-Controlled Trial. In: Program and Abstracts of the 2018 Annual Meeting of the American Association for the Study of Liver Diseases; November 9-13, 2018; San Francisco, California. Abstract LB 4

[35] Harrison FA, Guy CD, Bashir M, et al. In a Placebo-Controlled 36-Week Phase 2 Trial, treatment with Mgl-3196 compared to placebo results in significant reductions in hepatic fat (MRI-PDFF), liver enzymes, fibrosis biomarkers, atherogenic lipids, and improvement in NASH on serial liver biopsy. In: Program and Abstracts of the 2018 Annual Meeting of the American Association for the Study of Liver Diseases; November 9-13, 2018; San Francisco, California. Abstract 14

[36] Charlton MR, Lai M, Noureddin M. GS-0976, a liver-targeted acetyl-coa carboxylase (ACC) inhibitor, reduces plasma acylcarnitines in patients with nonalcoholic steatohepatitis (NASH). In: Program and abstracts of the 2018 Annual Meeting of the American Association for the Study of Liver Diseases; November 9-13, 2018; San Francisco, California. Abstract 1741

[37] Ratziu O, Ladron-De-Guevara L, Safadine R. One year results of the Global Phase 2b Randomized Placebo-Controlled Arrest Trial of Aramchol, a Stearoyl CoADesaturase Inhibitor, in patients with NASH. In: Program and abstracts of the 2018 Annual Meeting of the American Association for the Study of Liver Diseases; November 9-13, 2018; San Francisco, California. Abstract LB 5

[38] Newsome PN, Harrison SA, Rasmussen S. The Effect of semaglutide on liver enzymes in subjects with obesity and elevated alanine aminotransferase: Data from a randomized Phase 2 Trial. In: Program and abstracts of the 2018 Annual Meeting of the American Association for the Study of Liver Diseases; November 9-13, 2018; San Francisco, California. Abstract 105

[39] Lassailly G et al. Bariatric surgery reduces features of nonalcoholic steatohepatitis in morbidly obese patients. Gastroenterology. 2015;**149**:379-388

[40] Bower G et al. Bariatric surgery and non-alcoholic fatty liver disease: A systematic review of liver biochemistry and histology. Obesity Surgery. 2015;**25**:2280-2289

Section 2

Management of Cirrhosis and Its Complications

Chapter 4

Formation of Systemic Changes Features with Fatal Complications of Metabolic Syndrome and Chronic Diffuse Liver Diseases

Boris Fishman, Vladimir Kulikov, Svetlana Butrimova, Spartak Turmakhanov, Mikhail Yukhno, Irina Prozorova, Pavel Starikov, Oksana Lole and Vyacheslav Zurabov

Abstract

Chronic liver disease at initial stages often occurs with no symptoms or with very non-specific symptoms, so timely diagnosis of chronic liver disease is of great importance, and there are significant difficulties involved therein. Not being able to diagnose the hepatic disease early, difficulties with the management of the disease and treatment arise. Different aspects of the clinical and laboratory evaluation may be of assistance in providing an early diagnosis, ranging from laboratory tests, to ultrasound, to EGD, and to rheohepatography (not used that frequently) among others. Stages of hepatitis affect the hepatic and general symptoms, and morphological changes in liver tissue are presented and discussed, followed by a section devoted to hepatic encephalopathy (HE) and how it is influenced by cerebral hemodynamics and state of liver cirrhosis (LC).

Keywords: liver, chronic hepatitis, liver cirrhosis, chronic diffuse liver disease, hepatic encephalopathy

1. Introduction

Chronic hepatitis (CH) and liver cirrhosis (LC), especially the latter, are the most common cause of portal hypertension (PH), leading to changes in the functional ability of the affected organ, which is manifested by corresponding changes in blood biochemical parameters. At the same time, among the many clinical manifestations of the disease, there is no symptomatology pathogenic for these conditions, which allows for a timely diagnosis. That leads to the difficulties of early detection of the transition of the inflammatory process of the liver to the cirrhosis, and the possibility of initiating timely treatment.

In patients of different age groups with liver cirrhosis of viral etiology of classes A, B, and C according to Child-Pugh, chronic hepatic encephalopathy of all stages can occur against the background of dyscirculatory disorders with the development of chronic cirrhosis (LC) with the rapid disability of patients. In recent decades, studies have been conducted on the effect of LC on the severity of hepatic encephalopathy (HE), etiology, stages of the disease, and psychological characteristics of the personality [1–4]. In modern approaches to the treatment of LC, it is necessary to take into account the etiological factor, the reduction of pathogenetic reactions that support the activity of the process, prevention of progression of cirrhosis, treatment of symptoms, and complications of the disease such as portal hypertension, HE, ascites, ascites-peritonitis, and hepatorenal syndrome. HE can be subclinical in nature, and mortality among patients is up to 10% and is mostly associated with comorbidities, and not with complications of portal hypertension [5–8]. Therefore, the assessment of the degree of HE and the corresponding individualized approach to each patient in terms of the selection of therapy can significantly reduce its stage, which also improves the quality of life of patients [9, 10]

1.1 Materials and research methods

The most common methods of laboratory diagnosis of chronic diffuse liver disease (CDLD) are biochemical analysis of blood, the study of coagulation with the assessment of coagulation, anticoagulation systems, and special tests to determine some of the complications of the underlying disease. The case of active and complicated course of the disease can be obtained from a general blood test. Indicators of coagulation and blood rheology are important, excluding in the postoperative period a number of serious complications due to impaired microcirculation can develop and including acute hepatocellular insufficiency, gastrointestinal bleeding, and even with inactive liver cirrhosis.

1.2 Materials and research methods used for assessing hepatic encephalopathy

One hundred seven patients (87 (81.3%) men and 20 (18.7%) women) with viral etiology LC were examined: HBV infection (n = 35.1%), HCV infection (n = 46.1%), and infection HBV + HCV (n = 18.8%) aged from 30 to 69 years (average age was 57.3 ± 4.6 years). According to the compensation stages by Child-Pugh LC, the patients were divided into three groups: the first group (n = 35) consisted of Class A LC patients, the second group (n = 37) consisted of Class B patients, and the third group (n = 35) included patients with Class C LC. To confirm the diagnosis of LC and its etiology and stage of compensation and complications, the clinical picture and history of the disease were studied; a complex of clinical, laboratory and instrumental diagnostic methods was conducted. To match the fibrosis index and the LC for METAVIR and ISHAK, a classification counting scale (Bonacini) was used. Patients with cardiac arrhythmias and hormonal status were excluded from the study, without heart defects and an increase in blood pressure above stage III.

Clinical diagnosis of HE, assessment of its severity, and basic and additional instrumental studies were conducted in accordance with the recommendations of the working group of the 11th World Congress of Gastroenterologists. Evaluation of the stages of HE was carried out according to a descriptive scale of West-Haven symptoms and Reitan test (number connection test). Ultrasound diagnosis of cerebral hemodynamics was performed using the PHILIPS EPIQ 7G ultrasound machine (USA) using the W. J. Zwiebel, J. S. Pellerito method (2010). Diagnostics of brain blood flow included the study of blood flow parameters in the internal carotid (ICA) and middle cerebral arteries (MCA) of the first order of both hemispheres, maximal, minimal, and average BFV; contralateral asymmetry of the mean BFV; carbon-dependent blood flow indicators (RI and PI); cerebral perfusion pressure; reactivity of blood flow; cerebrovascular blood reserve; cerebrovascular reactivity index; and vasomotor reactivity, were determined by the functional reserve of the connecting arteries of the circle of Willis Matas sample. To study the function of the heart in LC, echocardiography was performed in the M-modal and two-dimensional modes according to the standard method of the American Association of Echocardiography. In 15.9% of cases, autopsy material served as the object of research of the abdominal cavity and brain. For the differential diagnosis of LC and its complications, CT, MRI, FGDS, Reitan's combination test, and electroencephalography were performed.

The study of the parameters of cerebral hemodynamics with LC of classes A, B, and C consisted of several stages. At the first stage, the parameters of central hemodynamics were studied. The central element in this question was the study of the systolic function of the left ventricle. At the second stage, the parameters of cerebral hemodynamics were studied. The results of the average values of blood flow parameters and intima-media complex (IMC) thickness in the internal carotid arteries with LC of classes A, B, and C were analyzed. In addition, the presence of hemisphere asymmetry was associated with the development of dyscirculatory disorders, confirmed by neuroimaging and autopsy of the brain. Thus, in the prospective observation, the autopsy material of the brain served as confirmation of the comorbidity of HE and dyscirculatory disorders from minimal to irreversible with the LC.

All patients with clinical and instrumental signs of chronic HE and cerebrovascular insufficiency were given a psychometric test of Reitan for the connection of numbers.

Processing of the obtained clinical and laboratory and instrumental data was carried out using the criteria of parametric and nonparametric statistics. The magnitude of the distribution of the Gauss density was estimated from the values of the interquartile range. The correlation matrix method was used to determine the degree of interrelation between individual signs. Statistical processing of the material obtained was carried out using the program Stat Soft Statistica, version 10.0.

2. Chronic hepatitis of minimal activity

The clinical picture of patients with minimal activity CH was characterized by a paucity of symptoms. The majority of patients (21) had an asymptomatic course of the disease. The admission of patients to the hospital was associated with symptoms of chronic cholecystitis or the presence of changes in the biochemical blood tests detected during the preventive examination. In some cases, treatment was associated with the appearance of some symptoms of asthenic and dyspeptic syndrome in individuals who considered themselves practically healthy. However, some patients complained of weakness (31.4%) and nausea (23.4%).

Careful collection of anamnesis showed that 66.2% (131) of the patients previously had AVH, 15.6% (31) had contact with patients with AVH, 12.1% (24) shortly before the disease underwent surgery and blood transfusion or long-term (more than 1 month) received intramuscular injections, and only 12 patients pointed to alcohol abuse.

In patients with chronic hepatitis (**Tables 1** and **2**), with minimal degree of activity, no statistically significant expansion of the diameter and cross-sectional area of the portal and splenic veins was compared with the control group.

There were also no statistically significant changes in the maximum and volumetric blood flow velocities through the portal and splenic veins with pulsed-wave Doppler sonography.

An increase in portal pressure primarily affects the volume velocity of the blood flow in the portal and then in the splenic veins, depending on its size. So, at the level of portal pressure up to 128.3–134.3 mm H_2O, a further increase in pressure in the

Indicators	CH of minimal activity (n = 207)		M ± SD in patients of control group (n = 40)	p
	Limits of variation	M ± SD		
Inner diameter, mm	9.0–13.0	10.71 ± 1.25	10.22 ± 0.71	>0.05
Cross-sectional area, sq. cm.	0.64–1.33	0.91 ± 0.05	0.83 ± 0.03	>0.05
Max BFV, cm/s	18.2–25.0	21.63 ± 1.56	21.63 ± 2.71	>0.05
BVF, ml/min.	686.3–1910.3	1161.91 ± 341.19	1075.8 ± 83.61	>0.05
Portal vein pressure, mm H_2O	98.3–164.3	123.3 ± 10.49	113.0 ± 4.41	>0.05

p—Statistical significance of the difference between control group and patients with chronic hepatitis.

Table 1.
Results of hemodynamic studies in the portal vein in patients with chronic hepatitis of minimal activity (M ± SD).

Indicators	CH of minimal activity (n = 207)		M ± SD in patients of control group (n = 40)	p
	Limits of variation	M ± SD		
Inner diameter, mm	6.0–8.0	6.63 ± 0.69	6.41 ± 0.61	>0.05
Cross-sectional area, sq. cm.	0.28–0.51	0.37 ± 0.02	0.33 ± 0.02	>0.05
Max BFV, cm/s	17.0–22.2	18.94 ± 0.97	19.22 ± 2.23	>0.05
BVF, ml/min.	274.3–539.6	379.51 ± 74.33	345.41 ± 34.62	>0.05

p—Statistical significance of the difference between control group and patients with chronic hepatitis.

Table 2.
Results of hemodynamic studies in the splenic vein with chronic hepatitis of minimal activity (M ± SD).

portal vein to 140.3–146.3 mm H_2O leads to initial changes in hemodynamics in the splenic vein.

Echographic signs of chronic cholecystitis with calculi of various sizes were found in 51.5% of patients.

CT scan, performed in 15.2% of patients, also showed no changes in the liver, with the exception of 60% of patients with chronic cholecystitis, where gallbladder calculi were visualized.

Radiocontrast study in eight (24.2%) patients revealed a diffusely uneven distribution of radiopharmaceuticals in the liver at normal sizes and even and clear contours of the organ.

Esophagogastroduodenoscopy in 24.4% of patients found superficial, in 21.2% atrophic, and in 3% subatrophic gastritis, in 21.2% duodenitis, in 12% duodenogastric, and in 15% gastroesophageal reflux, in some cases with erosive esophagitis.

Thus, the clinical diagnosis of minimal activity CH is based on a thorough collection of anamnesis, clarification of complaints, clinical symptoms, and laboratory data, which allows to establish a clinical diagnosis and determine the tactics of further research and treatment by the first day after admission. The information content of noninvasive additional research methods in patients of this group is extremely low. In this regard, morphological study is the most objective and informative diagnostic method.

A histological study conducted in 16 patients showed that 12 of them have a morphological picture of chronic persistent hepatitis, including 7 patients with chronic calculous cholecystitis.

Biopsy in this category of patients is very problematic, due to the frequent rejection of patients from the study, due to the invasiveness of the technique. At the same time, we consider it unnecessary to conduct histological studies on a universal basis, limiting the indications for its implementation only to those who need histological monitoring of the effectiveness of the treatment or surgical intervention, due to the long-term, uncorrected conservative therapy, and activation of the pathological process in the liver. In other cases, the activity of the pathological process should be determined by the level of transaminases (an increase in the ALT level to three norms).

3. Chronic hepatitis of moderate activity

The clinical manifestation in 39 patients with moderately active chronic hepatitis was different from the previous group by more intense symptoms than in the previous group. Most patients (30) were admitted to the clinic due to the existing symptoms of abdominal pain and dyspeptic, asthenic, and hemorrhagic syndromes. Twenty-three patients complained of pain (9) and severity (14) in the right hypochondrium, especially after an error in diet or exercise. In nine of them, the pain was paroxysmal. Six patients indicated nausea and vomiting (3) after ingestion of fatty foods, 7 patients indicated disorders of the stool, 6 patients indicated irritability, 14 patients indicated weakness, 7 patients indicated decreased performance, and 3 patients indicated bleeding from the nose and gums.

According to case records it turned out that 15 patients had previous AVH, 3 of them received hormonal therapy due to severe disease, 5 pointed to jaundice of unknown etiology, 6 contact with AVH patients, and 4 undergone surgery, blood transfusion, or prolonged (up to 1 month) intramuscular injections.

The general condition was assessed in 25 patients as satisfactory and in 14, moderate. Reduced nutrition occurred in 15 patients, single telangiectasia on the upper half of the chest in 4 patients. Yellow skin extinguishing and icteric sclera were observed in eight, palmar erythema in five patients. Visually abdominal distension was determined in four patients. On palpation, in 26 patients, an enlarged liver was protruded, projecting 2–3 cm from under the edge of the right costal arch. In 23 of them its compaction and tenderness was determined. The spleen in six patients was slightly enlarged; its lower pole was felt at the edge of the left costal arch without any subjective sensations.

Hypochromic anemia of grade 1 occurred in grade 7, grade 2, and grade 6, moderate transient thrombocytopenia in seven, and accelerated ESR in 22 patients. However, when recalculating the peripheral blood indices for the total number of patients with moderately active chronic gastritis, a moderate decrease in the number of red blood cells was obtained with relatively normal values of other peripheral blood indices. Evaluation of the functional state of the liver using a complex of biochemical research methods showed the depression of its function, which was expressed by a significant increase in bilirubin (58.1 ± 1.4 mmol/l) fractions of aminotransferases more than three standards (ALT, 2.27 ± 0.06; AST, 1.17 ± 0.06 mmol/h l). Dysproteinemia was observed (albumin 49.1 ± 0.89% and globulins 23.3 ± 0.35%), with a decrease in albumin/globulin coefficient (A/G ratio) to 0.96, with relatively normal indicator total protein levels.

In patients with chronic hepatitis of moderate degree of activity, the contours of the liver were even in only 154 (74.4%) patients, and the pointed edge of the liver was found in 169 (81.6%) patients. The echogenicity of the parenchyma is irregularly increased in 197 (80.7%) patients. In 143 (69.1%) patients, the phenomenon of "distal attenuation" of ultrasound was observed, while the oblique size of the right lobe of the liver was more than 160 mm. In addition, 28 (13.5%) patients with chronic hepatitis had abdominal lymphadenopathy at the gate of the liver.

In patients with chronic hepatitis of moderate activity of the inflammatory process (**Tables 3** and **4**), expansion of the portal vein diameter and, accordingly, an increase in its cross-sectional area against a background of pressure increase in it were noted. At the same time, there was no statistically significant increase in the internal diameter and cross-sectional area of the splenic vein; although in some patients, there was a change in both signs indicating increased portal pressure.

Doppler study of the blood flow in the portal vein did not show a statistically significant decrease in the maximum and increase in the volumetric flow rate. From the data presented in **Table 4**, it is also clear that signs of hemodynamic disturbances are observed in the splenic vein, which coincide in their direction with those in the portal vein, but quantitatively these changes are not so significant ($p > 0.05$).

Indicators	CH of moderate activity (n = 23)		M ± SD in patients of control group (n = 40)	p
	Limits of variation	M ± SD		
Inner diameter, mm	11.0–14.0	12.81 ± 1.11	10.2 ± 0.71	<0.05
Cross-sectional area, sq. cm.	0.95–1.54	1.29 ± 0.04	0.83 ± 0.03	<0.05
Max BFV, cm/s	16.1–23.2	18.92 ± 1.72	21.6 ± 2.71	<0.05
BVF, ml/min.	686.7–1898.1	1257.51 ± 355.23	1075.8 ± 83.61	<0.05
Portal vein pressure, mm H_2O	145.6–190.9	164.4 ± 9.34	113.0 ± 4.41	<0.05

p—Statistical significance of the difference between control group and patients with chronic hepatitis.

Table 3.
Results of hemodynamic studies in the portal vein in patients with chronic hepatitis of moderate activity (M ± SD).

Indicators	CH of moderate activity (n = 23)		M ± SD in patients of control group (n = 40)	p
	Limits of variation	M ± SD		
Inner diameter, mm	6.0–9.0	7.11 ± 0.83	6.4 ± 0.61	>0.05
Cross-sectional area, sq. cm.	0.28–0.64	0.41 ± 0.03	0.33 ± 0.02	>0.05
Max BFV, cm/s	15.2–20.1	17.81 ± 0.94	19.2 ± 2.23	>0.05
BVF, ml/min.	280.2–608.3	402.01 ± 84.41	345.4 ± 34.62	>0.05

p—Statistical significance of the difference between control group and patients with chronic hepatitis.

Table 4.
Results of hemodynamic studies in the splenic vein in patients with chronic hepatitis of moderate activity (M ± SD).

It is noted that the increase in portal pressure to the level of 170.3–174.4 mm H_2O led to changes in hemodynamic parameters: diameter and linear and volumetric blood flow velocity in the portal vein. A further increase in portal pressure to 178.4–182.6 mm H_2O influenced the change in the above parameters of hemodynamics in the splenic vein. First of all, these changes concerned the diameter of the portal vein and the volumetric blood flow in the hepatoportal bed.

CT, as well as in the previous group of patients, was performed in a limited number of 42 patients (20.3%). In the study in addition to moderate hepatomegaly, changes in the parenchyma of the liver were not found. In 32 cases, along with an increase in the size of the liver, concrements of the gallbladder were detected.

Radiocontrast study performed in 39% of patients revealed a moderate increase in the size of the liver and, in 82% of cases, a diffuse decrease in the accumulative function of the organ. In 5% of cases there was a redistribution of the radiopharmaceutical in the spleen.

EGD was performed in 149 (72%) patients; in 69 of them inflammatory, changes of the upper digestive tract were found in the form of superficial (32), erosive gastritis, duodenitis (32), duodenogastric (1), and gastroesophageal (4) reflux.

Thus, patients with chronic hepatitis of moderate activity are characterized by the presence of more constant clinical and laboratory changes that characterize the patient's true state. In a similar situation, conducting additional noninvasive research methods (ultrasound and radiocontrast study) allows a certain part of patients to reveal data (a uniform increase in the size of the liver, changes in the parenchyma of the organ) characterizing the morpho-functional state of the affected organ.

Histological studies of liver tissue carried out in 28 patients, in order to detect the morphological state of the liver; 61% of the examined patients found a picture of chronic persistent (CPH), and 39% had chronic active hepatitis (CAH).

Morphological studies of patients with chronic CH activity are not only diagnostic and diagnostic but also tactical. More than 1/3 of the patients in this group have a histological picture of CAH, in which the treatment tactics is somewhat different than with CPH. Therefore, for the development of a pathogenetic-based surgical tactics for chronic hepatitis C, we consider it expedient to perform not only intraoperative but also preoperative liver biopsy.

4. Chronic hepatitis of severe activity

This group consisted of 171 patients with the most prominent clinical symptoms of severe disease. Complaints and manifestations of the disease included almost the entire clinical syndromology of CDLD. The majority of patients (84.2%) complained of pain or heaviness in the right hypochondrium and epigastrium (abdominal pain syndrome); 63.2% of patients complained of weakness and fatigue; 47.4% - reduction of working ability (asthenic syndrome); 58% - loss of appetite; 21% - weight loss; 21% - nausea; 15.8% - disorders of the stool and flatulence (dyspeptic syndrome); 15.8% - jaundice; 15.8% - pruritus; 15.8% - dark urine; 10.5% - bleeding from the nose and gums; 5.3% - subcutaneous hemorrhages; 5.3% - menorrhagia; 10.5% - dysmenorrhea (endocrine syndrome); 15.8% - increase in the size of the abdomen and decreased diuresis; 10.5% - leg swelling (edema-ascitic syndrome); 10.5% - by memory loss, drowsiness, and periods of disorientation in time and space; and 5.3% - improper behavior (encephalopathy syndrome). In 26.3% of patients, the appearance of the above complaints was accompanied by an increase in body temperature to 38–39°C.

Anamnestic data showed that 90 patients in the period from 4 months to 11 years ago had AVH, 18 of them received hormonal (prednisolone) therapy due to severe disease, 18 indicated episodes of jaundice of unknown etiology, 36 on contact with AVH patients, 18 for previous surgical interventions with transfusion of donor blood or long-term infusion and injection therapy, and 9 for taking antituberculosis drugs (rifampicin, isoniazid, streptomycin, and analogues of these drugs) for 1 year or more, according to suspected pulmonary tuberculosis.

Condition of 18 patients at admission to the clinic is regarded as satisfactory, 126 moderate, and 27 severe. Severity of the condition was due to the course of the underlying disease, as well as secondary changes from other organs. Severe jaundice occurred in 27 patients; in 9 of them with subcutaneous hemorrhages; in 18 patients with telangiectasias on the skin of the chest, shoulders, and face; and in 9 patients with urticaria on the face and neck. Yellowness of the skin and sclera was detected in 45 patients. And at 18 it was accompanied by skin itch, as evidenced by the traces of scratches that were present in these patients. Palmar erythema was found in 30 patients. Nutrition in 42 patients was reduced, and in 27 patient, there was pronounced weight loss. However, only nine patients indicated weight loss during the last 6 months.

According to 45 patients auscultation data, systolic murmur at the apex of the heart and at the Erb's point was heard. A moderate increase in the abdomen occurred in 36 patients. On palpation, 108 patients had hepatomegaly, and in 26 of them, the lower edge of the liver protruded more than 5 cm from under the edge of the right costal arch (along the midclavicular line to the right). The edge of the liver, as a rule, is rounded, the surface is smooth, and tissue is somewhat thickened and painful. In 18 cases, an enlarged, painful, slightly tense gallbladder was palpable. In 36 patients enlarged spleen was determined, tissue being compacted and painful on palpation. In 18 of them, the lower pole of the organ emerged from under the edge of the left costal arch by 3–5 cm and in 9 by more than 6 cm. Free fluid in the abdominal cavity was detected in 11 patients with a severe course of the pathological process.

Patients in this group had hypochromic anemia, moderate thrombocytopenia (platelets less than 200,000), and accelerated ESR. Liver function was characterized by severe hyperbilirubinemia (total of 74.2 ± 8.2 mmol/l), mainly due to the direct fraction (49.7, 1.9), increased transaminase levels (AlAT, 2.67±0, 12; AsAT, 1.6 ± 0.15 mmol/h l), and in 7 (21%) dysproteinemia in the form of hypoalbuminemia (45.8 ± 0.53%) and hypergammaglobulinemia (25.9 ± 0.4%). Thymol test result tended to increase (9.0 ± 0.5 units), reaching 31 units in severe patients.

Ultrasound examination in all patients of this group revealed an increase in the size of the liver compared with the data of the previous group (**Table 5**). In patients with chronic hepatitis of high activity in 64 (37.4%) patients, the contours of the liver were lightly wavy; in 54 (31.6%) the edge of the liver was rounded. In 153 (89.5%) patients, the echogenicity of the liver parenchyma was unevenly elevated. The phenomenon of "distal attenuation" of ultrasound was detected in 134 (78.4%) patients, while the oblique size of the right lobe of the liver was more than 180 mm. In addition, 49 (28.78%) patients had lymphadenopathy in the gates of the liver, and 11 (6.4%) patients had a small amount of free fluid in the abdominal cavity, indicating the development of portal hypertension in these patients, which is not rare. It happens with the so-called "active" hepatitis at the height of the clinical and morphological manifestations of the disease.

A statistically significant enlargement of the liver in comparison with the control group was observed due to the total liver lobes: right to 186.13 ± 7.45 mm and 90.61 ± 6.81 mm and the caudate to 24.36±1.43 mm. The area of the spleen in this group of patients was up to 40.93±1.99 sq. cm.

Results presented in **Tables 6** and 7 rather convincingly indicate that patients with chronic hepatitis of a high degree of inflammatory activity show significant disorders of hepatic hemodynamics, manifested by a relatively high level of portal

Indicators Size, mm	**CH of severe activity (n = 23)**		**M ± SD in patients of control group (n = 40)**	**p**
	Limits of variation	**M ± SD**		
Liver				
Oblique size of the right lobe	120.0–205.0	186.13 ± 7.45	137.81 ± 1.79	>0.05
Anteroposterior size of the left lobe	66.0–114.0	90.61 ± 6.81	55.72 ± 1.87	>0.05
Anteroposterior size of the caudate lobe	21.0–30.0	17.63 ± 1.8	17.63 ± 1.83	>0.05
Spleen				
Area, sq. cm	31.9–45.1	40.93 ± 1.99	31.84 ± 1.49	>0.05

p—Statistical significance of the difference between control group and patients with chronic hepatitis.

Table 5.
Liver and spleen dimensions in patients with chronic hepatitis of severe activity (M ± SD).

Indicators	**CH of severe activity (n = 23)**		**M ± SD in patients of control group (n = 40)**	**p**
	Limits of variation	**M ± SD**		
Inner diameter, mm	12.0–15.0	13.79 ± 1.01	10.22 ± 0.71	>0.05
Cross-sectional area, sq. cm.	1.13–1.77	1.51 ± 0.06	0.83 ± 0.04	>0.05
Max BFV, cm/s	15.1–20.0	17.33 ± 1.33	21.63 ± 2.71	>0.05
BVF, ml/min.	772.3–1863.9	1327.73 ± 315.81	1075.81 ± 83.61	>0.05
Portal vein pressure, mm H_2O	169.9–212.4	193.4 ± 9.47	113.0 ± 4.41	>0.05

p—Statistical significance of the difference between control group and patients with chronic hepatitis.

Table 6.
Results of hemodynamic studies in the portal vein in patients with chronic hepatitis of severe activity (M ± SD).

pressure and dilatation of the portal and splenic veins without changing the velocity parameters of blood flow in them.

It is noted that the increase in portal pressure to the level of 185.5–197.2 mm H_2O leads to a change in hemodynamic parameters: diameter and linear and volumetric blood flow velocity in the portal (mainly) and splenic veins. At first, volumetric blood flow velocity increases due to pressure in the above veins.

Thus, in patients with chronic hepatitis, there were changes in the echographic parameters of the liver and spleen, as well as the parameters of portal hemodynamics, depending on the degree of development of the cytolytic syndrome.

Radiocontrast study performed in 108 patients found an increase in the size of the liver, and in 9 of them there was a diffuse uneven accumulation of radiopharmaceuticals in the liver and its redistribution into the spleen (in 36). In 45 cases, these changes are estimated as CH transition to liver cirrhosis.

Indicators	CH of severe activity (n = 23)		M ± SD in patients of control group (n = 40)	p
	CI (25–75%)	SD		
Inner diameter, mm	7.0–10.0	8.06 ± 0.91	6.41 ± 0.61	>0.05
Cross-sectional area, sq. cm.	0.44–0.81	0.59 ± 0.06	0.33 ± 0.02	>0.05
Max BFV, cm/s	15.1–19.02	16.78 ± 0.90	19.22 ± 2.23	>0.05
BVF, ml/min.	307.26–69,631.9	453.96 ± 99.08	345.41 ± 34.62	>0.05

p—Statistical significance of the difference between control group and patients with chronic hepatitis.

Table 7.
Results of hemodynamic studies in the splenic vein in patients with chronic hepatitis of severe activity (M ± SD).

EGD in 153 patients found inflammatory changes in the esophagus, stomach, and duodenum. At the same time, 18 of them revealed superficial, 72 erosive gastritis, 27 duodenitis, 36 duodenogastric, 27 duodenogastric, and 77 gastroesophageal refluxes; 27 patients with this group showed varicose veins of the lower third of the esophagus grades I–II.

A pronounced clinical manifestation of the disease allows a more correct assessment of the patient's condition and a correct preliminary diagnosis and determination of the correct diagnostic and therapeutic tactics. Ultrasound, radiocontrast study, and EGD in patients with chronic hepatitis of severe activity show an important diagnostic value and make it possible to identify some signs of a complicated course of the disease, which are not determined in a routine clinical study. Radiocontrast study in five patients, long before the liver biopsy, established signs of transition of CH to cirrhosis.

Pre- and intraoperative morphological studies of the liver in 16 patients of this group, in 7% of cases, established a histological picture of CPH, in 82% CAH, and in 11% CAH with transition to LC.

Thus, in the diagnosis of chronic hepatitis of severe activity, great importance, in addition to clinical, laboratory, and morphological data, is acquired by using modern noninvasive research methods, which provide sufficient information for correct diagnosis. In our opinion, in the diagnosis of CH of severe activity, it is necessary to give preference to noninvasive ultrasound and radiocontrast methods and resort to the use of invasive (biopsy, laparoscopy, etc.) ones only in exceptional cases, because any active interventions in this category of patients can lead to decompensation of the disease.

5. Cerebral hemodynamic influence on the current and prediction of hepatic encephalopathy

In recent decades, studies have been conducted on the effects of cirrhosis of the liver (LC) on the severity of chronic hepatic encephalopathy (HE), etiology, stage, and psychological characteristics of the personality [11–14]. HE can be subclinical, and the mortality rate among patients is up to 10% and is mostly associated with comorbidities, and not with complications of PG [15–18]. That is why the assessment of the degree of HE and the corresponding individualized approach to each patient in terms of the selection of therapy can significantly reduce the degree of encephalopathy, which also improves the quality of life of patients [19, 20]. In many pathological conditions, the occurrence of encephalopathy signals a disorder of brain metabolism, based on the formation of which is a violation of the blood-brain barrier, the action of toxic substances, cerebral ischemia, cerebral hypoxia, the formation of endotoxins, and neurotransmitter disorders. In most cases, there is a combination of several pathophysiological mechanisms. And those, in turn, may lead to clinical picture of encephalopathy with cognitive, emotional, and motor impairment. However, despite numerous experimental and clinical studies of HE, the mechanism of its development remains controversial and controversial [21–24]. The purpose of this study is to assess the characteristics of cerebral hemodynamics in the extra- and intracranial sections with LC of viral etiology of classes A, B, and C according to Child-Pugh to improve the optimization of early diagnosis of complications of encephalopathy at various stages of its development.

It has been established that with an increase in the stage of hepatic encephalopathy, an increase in hemispheric asymmetry of blood flow in the middle cerebral arteries and in the time of the Reitan test is observed. The minimum time for connecting numbers during the test was noted at stage 1 of HE without comorbidity with circulatory encephalopathy (DE), the maximum with HE stage 3 in combination with DE stage 3.

Matrix analysis showed that, first, with an increase in the stages of hepatic encephalopathy, a statistically significant increase in the time to perform the Reitan test was observed. Secondly, the influence of the DE stages on the course of the HE stages is ambiguous, the minimum during stage I of the HE and the maximum with the HE of stage III. Thus, a statistically significant increase in the time of the Reitan test is recorded at stage I HE only in combination with stage III DE, at stage II HE, stage III DE, and stage III HE with any stage DE. When studying the characteristics of the relationship between the hemispheric asymmetry of the BFV in the MCA and the stages of HE, it was found that there is a fairly clear correlation between the hemisphere asymmetry of the blood flow in the MCA and the stages of the HE. Thus, with increasing stage of HE, hemispheric asymmetry of blood flow in MCA increases: the smallest hemisphere asymmetry of blood flow in MCA is observed with LC with clinical manifestations of HE of stages I–II and the greatest with HE of stages III–IV.

From the obtained results, it follows that the change in cerebral hemodynamics in patients with LC is noted already at the level of the extracranial section of the carotid arteries. The presence of age-related changes in the arteries, such as intimal thickening before the formation of atherosclerotic plaques of different height and length with the formation of stenosis, tortuosity of the vessels led to hemisphere asymmetry of blood flow in them from 25.1 ± 2.42 to 39.5 ± 7.94% with the dynamics of the statistical significance of this parameter in comparison with the norm from $p = 0.006936$ to $p = 0.000003$ for LC of classes A and C, respectively.

Functional disorders of cerebral hemodynamics at the level of the intracranial section manifested changes in blood flow velocity characteristics, lability of vascular resistance indices, hemispheric asymmetry of the blood flow, and decrease in the functional reserve of the connective arteries of the Willis circle. Against the background of atherosclerotic changes in the vascular wall and the lability of vascular resistance, there were large variations in the interquartile ranges of the velocity parameters of the blood flow and hemisphere asymmetry in the MCA with a general tendency of their medians to increase, which did not contradict the studies of other authors [25]. So, depending on the stage of compensation of the LC, there was a general tendency for the ACK (max) to increase from 110.7 ± 9.21 to 119.2 + 10.03 cm/s, ACK (min) from 48.5 = 9.76 up to 52.1 ± 10.95 cm/s, ASK (mean) from 69.6 ± 8.45 to 74.1—11 × 57 cm/s, and hemisphere asymmetry ASA (mean) from 24.9 ± 9.51 up to 33.9 ± 10.51 with LC of classes A and C, respectively. At the same time, it should be noted that there is a rather clear correlation between the stages of HE and hemisphere asymmetry of blood flow ($r = 0.495$). So, with increasing stage of HE, hemispheric asymmetry of blood flow along the MCA increases, caused, in our opinion, on the one hand by atherosclerosis, on the other by the lability of vascular resistance due to vasoconstrictive substances (nitric oxide, endothelin-1), whose concentration in the blood often increases with LC and atherosclerosis, which has been confirmed elsewhere [26, 27]. At the same time, the co-dependent indicators of vascular resistance had a clear downward trend depending on the degree of compensation of the LC. The dynamics of the statistical significance of this parameter in comparison with the norm for RI became reliable from $p = 0.245844$ to $p = 0.002776$ and PI from 0.071383 to 0.012336 with LC of classes A and C, respectively.

When conducting a comparative analysis of the blood flow velocity in MCA, two types of blood flow were identified—hypokinetic and hyperkinetic. Thus, with class C LC, in 21.4% of cases, the hyperkinetic type of blood flow was observed and which probably had a compensatory mechanism. In LC, damage occurs to the endothelial cells of the hepatic sinusoids, and the latter leads to a significant increase in the level of endothelin. With liver damage and the development of portal hypertension, the production of intrahepatic nitric oxide decreases, which leads to its imbalance. It should be noted that the known mechanisms of participation of endothelial dysfunction can be distinguished by the suppression of the excretion or inactivation of endothelial NO synthase and a decrease in the synthesis of NO, due to an increase in the level of cytokines and TNF-a, which suppress the synthesis of nitric oxide. During the formation of portal hypertension, the process of separation of the organ and the general blood flow is observed due to the development of an imbalance between vasodilating and vasoconstrictive substances. The release of vasoactive substances (histamine, serotonin), circulating vasodilators into the blood from damaged hepatocytes, leads to generalized vasodilation and a decrease in vascular resistance, which was confirmed in [28–31].

The data obtained by us indicate disorders in endothelium-dependent vasodilation and the vasomotor function of the endothelium in LC at various stages of compensation and are to a certain extent confirmed in [32–36]. Hemodynamics in the brain at a constant level was possible due to the normal functioning of the autoregulation mechanism, which ensured an unchanged level of the cerebral blood flow in the form of vasodilatation or vasoconstriction. At the same time, in the beyond vasodilation, the phenomenon of "sausage string" with segmental dilatation of arterioles may occur, against the background of which there is a danger of blood breakthrough into the brain tissue and the development of acute disorders of cerebral circulation. In the prospective observation, the autopsy material of the brain served as confirmation of this phenomenon and the development of dyscirculatory disorders from minimal to irreversible in LC.

6. Conclusion

Chronic hepatic encephalopathy due to LC with a frequency of up to 75% of cases can occur in comorbidity with dyscirculatory disorders from minimal to irreversible, which aggravates the clinical course of hepatic encephalopathy.

The effect of dyscirculatory disorders on the clinical course of the stages of hepatic encephalopathy is ambiguous. The minimal effect is observed at stage I of hepatic encephalopathy, the maximum at hepatic encephalopathy of stage III in comorbidity with the stages of dyscirculatory encephalopathy. The degree of cognitive and dyscirculatory disorders is interrelated with the stages of compensation for cirrhosis of the liver. With dyscirculatory disorders and a decrease in the stage of compensation for cirrhosis of the liver, there is an increase in the degree of cognitive impairment from the ability to logical thinking and attention to disorientation in time and space.

The Reitan test duration is more than 200 s, the presence of hemispheric asymmetry of the blood flow is more than 40%, and the decrease in the velocity parameters of the blood flow and vascular resistance indices in the basins of the middle cerebral arteries below the reference values are associated with an unfavorable prognosis of hepatic encephalopathy due to the possibility of the sausage-string phenomenon with the risk of development acute disorders of cerebral circulation of hemorrhagic type, development of venous stasis, and swelling in the brain.

Conflict of interest

All authors have not disclosed potential conflicts of interest regarding the content of this paper. The research was made in the frame of the work plan of Post Diploma Education and Polyclinic Therapy of NovSU and budget financing of city treatment and prevention institutions.

Author details

Boris Fishman[1*], Vladimir Kulikov[2], Svetlana Butrimova[3], Spartak Turmakhanov[1], Mikhail Yukhno[1,4], Irina Prozorova[1], Pavel Starikov[4], Oksana Lole[4] and Vyacheslav Zurabov[1]

1 Yaroslav-the-Wize Novgorod State University, Institute of Medical Education, Veliky Novgorod, Russia

2 Ulyanovsk State University, Ulyanovsk, Russia

3 Regional Clinical Hospital, Veliky Novgorod, Russia

4 Central City Clinical Hospital, Veliky Novgorod, Russia

*Address all correspondence to: fishman@mxc.ru

References

[1] Batskov SS, Zhdanov VP. Zhuravlev YF. Materialy XVII nauchno-prakticheskoy konferentsii vrachey OL LVO. L., 1989. pp. 11-12. (in Russian) [Бацков С.С., Жданов В.П., Журавлев Ю.Ф. Значение эхографии печени и желчевыводящих путей в диагностике вирусных гепатитов. Материалы XVII научно-практической конференции врачей ОЛ ЛВО. – Л., 1989. – С.11-12.]

[2] Batskov SS. Ultrazvukovoi Metod issledovaniia v gastroenterologii. SPb., 1995. S. 188 (in Russian) [Бацков С.С. Ультразвуковой метод исследования в гастроэнтерологии. – СПб., 1995. – С.188]

[3] Batskov SS, Gordiyenko AV. Klinicheskaia gepatologiia I pankreatologiia. SPRb.: V MedA; 1997. p. 119, 298 (in Russian) [Бацков С.С., Гордиенко А.В. Клиническая гепатология и панкреатология.// СПРб.: В МедА. – 1997. – С.119, 298]

[4] Borisov NA, Ryzhkov VK, Gapchenko YM. Vestnik khirurgii. 1988;**4**:17-22 (in Russian) [Борисов Н.А., Рыжков В.К., Гапченко Е.М. //Вестник хирургии. – 1988. - №4. – С.17-22]

[5] Aprosina ZG. Chronicheskii aktivnii gepatit kak sistemnii zabolevaniia– M.: Medicina. 1981. p. 248 (in Russian) [Апросина З.Г. Хронический активный гепатит как системные заболевания. – М.: Медицина, 1981. – С.248]

[6] Blyuger AF, Novitskiy NN. Prakticheskaia gepatologiia. Riga; 1984. (in Russian) [Блюгер А.Ф., Новицкий Н.Н. Практическая гепатология. – Рига, 1984]

[7] Bulanov KI. Sostoianie gepatoportalnoi gemodinamiki pri cirroze pecheni s sindromom portalnoi gipertenzii M. 1990. pp. 18-20 (in Russian) [Буланов К.И. Состояние гепатопортальной гемодинамики при циррозе печени с синдромом портальной гипертензии. – М., 1990. – С.18-20]

[8] Vlakhov N, Boyeva S, Porushev D, Tomova Ye. Vozmoznost sonografii i radionuklidnoi scanografii v diagnostici ochagobich idiffuznich porageniq pechtni. Meditsinskaya Radiologiya. 1985;**30**(2):70-71 (in Russian) [Влахов Н., Боева С., Порушев Д., Томова Е. Возможность сонографии и радионуклидной сканографии в диагностике очаговых и диффузных поражений печени.//Медицинская радиология. – 1985. – Т.30. - №2. – С.70-71]

[9] Bisset R, Khan A. Differencialnii analiz pri ultrazvukovom obsltdovanii. Vitebsk. 1997. pp. 25-211 (in Russian) [Биссет Р., Хан А. Дифференциальный диагноз при абдоминальном ульт-развуковом исследовании.//Витебск. – 1997. – С.25-211]

[10] Blyuger AF. Klinicheskii problemi chronicheskogo gepatita. Klinicheskaya meditsina. 1980;**58**(9):15-22 (in Russian) [Блюгер А.Ф. Клинические проблемы хронического гепатита. Обзор.// Клиническая медицина. – 1980. – Т.58. - №9. – С.15-22]

[11] Golovanova EV. Gastroenterologiya. / Mechanizmi fibroobrazovanii pri chronicheskich zabolevaniach pecheni I vozmognosti antifibroticheskoi terapii. Gastroenterologiia. 2014;**8**:52-59 (in Russian) [Голованова Е.В. Механизмы фиброзообразования при хронических заболеваниях печени и возможности антифибротической терапии]

[12] Filippova LP, Beloborodova EI, Beloborodova EV, Alekseeva AS, Shepeleva EG. Kachestvo gizni bolnich cirrozom pecheni v zavisimosti ot tonusa vegetativnoi nervnoi sistemi. Byulleten sibirskoj mediciny. 2012;**4**:152-157 (in Russian) [Филиппова Л.П., Белобородова Э.И., Белобородова Е.В., Алексеева А.С., Шепелева Е.Г. Качество жизни больных циррозом печени в зависимости от тонуса вегетативной нервной системы. Бюллетень сибирской медицины. 2012. № 4. С. 152-157]

[13] Kutepov DE. Ocenka effektivnosti lechtnia pacientov c pechenochnoi encefalopatiei. Kazanskij medicinskij zhurnal. 2014;**4**:496-501 (in Russian) [Кутепов Д.Е. Оценка эффективности лечения пациентов с печеночной энцефалопатией Казанский медицинский журнал. 2014. № 4. С. 496-501]

[14] Nazyrov FG, Devyatov AV, Babadzhanov AH, Raimov SA. Osobennosti razvitiia I techenia oslognenii cirroza pecheni v zavisimosti ot etiologicheskogo faktora. Novosti hirurgii. 2013;**4**:45-50 (in Russian) [Назыров Ф.Г., Девятое А.В., Бабаджанов А.Х., Раимов С.А. Особенности развития и течения осложнений цирроза печени в зависимости от этиологического фактора Новости хирургии. 2013. № 4. С. 45-50]

[15] Horonko YV, Polyak MI, Shitikov IV, Dmitriev AV, Sarkisov AE, Mikryukov VA. Minimizacia riskov pri tranugularnom vnutri pechenochnom portosistemnom chuntirovanii u bolnich c portalnoi gipertenziei, vizvannoi cirrozom pecheni. Vestnik hirargicheskoj gastroenterologii. 2012;**4**:48-53 (in Russian) [Хоронько Ю.В., Поляк М.И., Шитиков И.В., Дмитриев А.В., СаркисовА.Э., Микрюков В.А. Минимизация рисков при трансъюгулярном внутри печеночном портосистемном шунтировании (tips/типс) у больных с портальной гипертензией, вызванной циррозом печени Вестник хирургической гастроэнтерологии. 2012. № 4. С. 48-53]

[16] Avdej GM, Kulesh SD, Shumskas MS, Nikonova LV, Avdey SA, Lukyaniuk TN, et al. Ocenka effektivnosti primenenia preparata tiocetam u bolnich s encefalopatiei raslichnogo geneza. Vestnik vosstanovitelnoj mediciny. 2014;**3**:5-6 (in Russian) [Авдей Г.М., Кулеш С.Д., Шумскас М.С., Никонова Л.В., Авдей С.А., Лукьянюк Т.Н. Полюхович Ю.И., Давыдчик Э.В. Оценка эффективности применения препарата тиоцетам у больных с энцефалопатией различного генеза Вестник восстановительной медицины. 2014. № 3. С. 5-6]

[17] Russkih AV, Fomin W. Pechenochnoi encefalopatiei I principi ee lechenia. Farmateka. 2012;**13**:94-97 (in Russian) [Русских А.В., Фомин В.В. Печеночная энцефалопатия и принципы ее лечения Фарматека. 2012. № 13. С. 94-97]

[18] Homazyuk TA, Berezuckij VI, Kryzhanovskaya SI, Novozhenina LI, Filenko EI. Pechenochnoi encefalopatiei: Vozmogna li medicinskaia reabilitaciia? Mesto I effektivnost tiocetama Narkologiia. Narkologiya. 2013;**10**: 65-68 (in Russian) [Хомазюк Т.А., Березуцкий В.И., Крыжановская СИ., Новоженина Л.И., Филенко Е.И. Печеночная энцефалопатия: возможна ли медицинская реабилитация? Место и эффективность тиоцетама Наркология. 2013. № 10. С. 65-68]

[19] Rejnyuk VL, Shefer TV, Krasnov KA, Ivnickij YY. Vliianie ciklofosfana I laktulozi na postuplenie ammiaka I

vechestv srednei mollekularnoi massi iz kichechnika v krov u kris. Byulleten eksperimentalnoj biologii i mediciny. 2012;**10**:455-458 (in Russian) [Рейнюк В.А., Шефер Т.В., Краснов К.А., Ивницкий Ю.Ю. Влияние циклофосфана и лактулозы на поступление аммиака и веществ средней молярной массы из кишечника в кровь у крыс Бюллетень экспериментальной биологии и медицины. 2012. № 10. С. 455-458]

[20] Pizova NV. Encefalopatiei v nevrologicheskoi practice. Spravochnik poliklinicheskogo vracha. 2014;**6**:30-35 (in Russian) [Пизова Н.В. Энцефалопатии в неврологической практике Справочник поликлинического врача. 2014. № 6. С. 30-35]

[21] Yakovenko EP, Yakovenko AV, Kagramanova AV, Pryanishnikova AS, Ivanov AN, Agafonova NA, et al. Sovremenii podchodi k terapii bolnich cirrozom pecheni. Farmateka. 2012;**13**:88-93 (in Russian) [Яковенко Э.П., Яковенко А.В., Каграманова А.В., Прянишникова А.С., Иванов А.Н., Агафонова Н.А., Волошейникова Т.В, Григорьева Ю.В. Современные подходы к терапии больных циррозом печени Фарматека. 2012. № 13. С. [88-93]

[22] Morozova TS, Grishina IF, Gurikova IA. Ocobennosti cerebralnoi gemodinamici u pcientov s chronicheskimi diffuznimi zabolevaniiami pecheni. Kazanskij medicinskij zhurnaL. 2014;**6**:859-865 (in Russian) [Морозова Т.С., Гришина И.Ф., Гурикова И.А. Особенности церебральной гемодинамики у пациентов с хроническими диффузными заболеваниями печени Казанский медицинский журнал. 2014. № 6. С. 859-865]

[23] Ardatskaya MD, Minushkin ON. Sovremennii podchodi k diagnostiki I lecheniu pechenochnoi encefalopatiei. Gastroenterologiya. 2012;**8**:41-47 (in Russian) [Ардатская М.Д., Минушкин О.Н. Современные подходы к диагностике и лечению печеночной энцефалопатии]

[24] Bueverov AO. Patogeneticheskie osnovi pechenochnoi encefalopatiei: focus na ammiak. Klinicheskie perspektivy v gastroenterology gepatologii. 2012;**6**:3-10 (in Russian) [Буеверов А.О. Патогенетические основы печеночной энцефалопатии: фокус на аммиак Клинические перспективы в гастроэнтерологии, гепатологии. 2012. № 6. С. 3-10.]

[25] Lelyuk SE, Lelyuk VG. Metodicheskie aspekty ultrazvukovogo issledovaniya cerebrovaskulyarnoj reaktivnosti v norme i pri ateroskleroticheskom porazhenii brahiocefalnyh arterij: uchebnoe posobie. Moscow: RMAPO; 2010. 31 p. (in Russian) [Лелюк С.Э., Лелюк В.Г. Методические аспекты ультразвукового исследования цереброваскулярной реактивности в норме и при атеросклеротическом поражении брахиоцефальных артерий: учебное пособие. М.: РМАПО, 2010. 31 с.]

[26] Mirodzhanov GK, Avezov SA, Giyasov MM, Abdullaeva ZM. Interleikin 6 I oksid azota v patogeneze portalnoi gipertenzii I dekompensaciicorroza pechtni. Klinicheskaya Medicina. 2012;**1**: 47-53 (in Russian) [Мироджанов Г.К., Авезов С.А., Гансов М.М., Абдуллаева З.М. Интерлейкин-6 и оксид азота в патогенезе портальной гипертензии и декомпенсации цирроза печени Клиническаямедицина. 2012. № 1. С. 47-53]

[27] Abclullaev RF, Bashhaliev AB, Kulieva AD, Gusejn-zade RR. Ocenka zavisimosti koncentracii endotelina-1 I magnia v krovi ot stepeni tagesti

ichemicheskoi bolezni serdca. Kazanskij medicmskij zhurnal. 2016;**4**:492-496 (in Russian) [Абдуллаев Р.Ф., Башхалиев А.Б., Кулиева А.Д., Гусейн-заде Р.Р. Оценка зависимости концентрации эндотелина-1 и магния в крови от степени тяжести ишемической болезни сердца Казанский медицинский журнал. 2016. № 4. С. 492-496.]

[28] Chen TA, Csao TY, Chen TA. Effect of intravenous albumin on endotoxin removal, cytokines, and nitric oxide production in patients with cirrhosis and spontaneous bacterial peritonitis. Scandinavian Journal of Gastroenterology. 2009;**44**:619-625

[29] Elsing C, Harenberg S, Stremmel W, Herrman T. Serum levels of soluble fas, nitric oxide and cytokines in acute decompensated cirrhotic patients. World Journal of Gastroenterology. 2007;**13**(3):421-425

[30] Anderson TJ. Nitric oxide, atherosclerosis and the clinical relevance of endothelial dysfunction. Heart Failure Reviews. 2003;**8**:71-86

[31] Kuksal AS, Koklu S, Ibis M, et al. Clinical features, serum interleukin-6, and interferon-gamma levels of 34 Turkish patients with hepatoportal sclerosis. Digestive Diseases and Sciences. 2007;**52**(12):3494-3497

[32] Tayanovskaya VY, Lelyuk VG, Kutuzova AB. Ultrazvukovaya ocenka cocudodvigatelnoq funkcii endotelia u lic,oblucytnnich v rslichnich dozach. Ultrazvukovaya i funkcionalnaya diagnostika. 2003;**1**:84-97 [Таяновская В.Ю., Лелюк В.Г., Кутузова А.Б. и др. Ультразвуковая оценка сосудодвигательной функции эндотелия у лиц, облученных в различных дозах Ультразвуковая и функциональная диагностика. 2003. № 1. С. 84-97]

[33] Kugiyama K, Ohgushi M, Mofoyama T, Sugiyama S, Ogawa H, Yoshimura M, et al. Nitric oxide-mediated flow-dependent dilation is impaired in coronary arteries in patients with coronary spastic angina. Journal of the American College of Cardiology. 1997;**30**:920-926

[34] Doronina NL. Sposob ocenki autoregulyacii mozgovogo krovoobrashheniya s pomoshhyu transkranialnoj stress-dopplerografii. Novosibirsk: Intermedika; 2001. 22 p. (in Russian) [Доронина Н.Л. Способ оценки ауторегуляции мозгового кровообращения с помощью транскраниальной стресс-допплерографии. Новосибирск: Интермедика, 2001. 22 p.]

[35] Svistov DV. Dopplerograficheskaya ocerika autoregulyatomogo rezerva sosudov golovnogo mozga v riorme i pri nejrohirurgicheskoj patologii. Otradnoe: Medsfera; 1998. 12 p. (in Russian) [Свистов Д.В. Допплерографическая оценка ауторегуляторного резерва сосудов головного мозга в норме и при нейрохирургической патологии. Отрадное: Медсфера, 1998. 12 с.]

[36] Chernikova IV, Kulikov VP, Kostyuchenko GI. Sosudodvigatelnaia funkcia endotelia u bolnich IBS s raslichnoi koncentraciei gomocecsteina v krovi. Ultrazvukovaya i funkcionalnaya diagnostika. 2006;**3**: 52-57 (in Russian) [Черникова И.В., Куликов В.П., Костюченко Г.И. Сосудодвигательная функция эндотелия у больных ишемической болезнью сердца с различной концентрацией гомоцистеина в крови Ультразвуковая и функциональная диагностика. 2006. № 3. С. 52-57.]

Chapter 5

Phytotherapy and Liver Disease

Lejla Čalkić

Abstract

Hepatoprotective agents are medicines or dietary supplements that are used as an adjunct to the treatment of acute and chronic viral hepatitis, liver cirrhosis, hepatocellular carcinoma prevention, as well as other liver diseases. Experiments on animals and cell cultures have shown that natural compounds can alleviate and prevent pathological changes in the liver. In the past few years, considerable attention has been paid to medicinal herbs with hepatoprotective, antioxidant, and immune properties. The plants contain numerous phytochemicals, including polyphenols, phenolic acids, coumarins, styles, tannins, lignans, and lignins. These compounds include silymarin, curcumin, picroside, kutkoside, phyllanthin, hypophyllanthin, glycyrrhizin, glycyrrhizin, berberine, luteolin, quercetin, coumarin derivatives (4-methylumbelliferone), and others. Many studies have been aimed at collecting data on some types of edible plants and fruits (grapefruit, cranberries, grapes, beets, cacti, chamomile, spirulina, propolis) that have shown hepatoprotective effects.

Keywords: plants, phytochemicals, dietary supplements, hepatitis, liver cirrhosis

1. Introduction

In liver disease treatment besides causal medicines, there are also antihepatotoxic, hepatotropic, and hepatoprotective agents. Hepatoprotective medicines or dietary supplements are used as an additional treatment for toxic liver damages, acute and chronic viral hepatitis, cirrhosis, and other liver diseases. There are numerous plants and traditional formulas used in liver disease treatments around the world.

2. Hepatoprotective plants and phytochemicals

Hepatoprotective chemicals are found in large number of medicinal herbs, out of which several were proven as very effective in various liver damages. Those compounds include silymarin, curcumin, picrorhiza and kutkoside, phyllanthin and hypophyllanthin, glycyrrhizin, berberine, luteolin, quercetin, and others [1]. Plants with polyphenol content (green tea) also indicate effectiveness in liver protection. It is determined that these compounds protect liver cells from various toxins, ischemic injuries, radioactive radiation, iron intoxication, and hepatotropic viruses [2]. The research suggests that these compounds increase protein synthesis, reduce tumor promoter's activity, stabilize mastocytes, modulate immune system, and have anti-inflammatory and anti-fibrotic effect. Many researches aimed at gathering information about some species of plants and fruits (grapefruit, cranberry, grapes, cacti, chamomile, and spirulina) which are often consumed and which have already shown hepatoprotective effects [3].

2.1 *Aloe vera* (lat. *Aloe barbadensis* M)

Aloe vera was named after botanist Miller who discovered and registered it in the registry of medicinal herbs. In the nature, it grows only in warm and dry climate areas, such as the Caribbean and Mexico. It has saber-like, pointy leaves which in its form remind of a rose and grow close to the ground. There are more than 250 species in the world, and only four have healing effect, among which predominantly is *Aloe vera* Barbadensis M. It was used as a medicine 6000 years ago in ancient Egypt, and back then it was known as "the herb of immortality." The most frequently used part of the plant is its gel, jelly-like mass from the inside of the leaf. *Aloe vera* has nutritious effect on every cell of the human organism, and because of its nutritional value and exceptional healing abilities, it is often called as "the queen of medicinal herbs." The gel contains more than 240 nutritious and healing ingredients: Vitamins A, B1, B2, B3, B6, B9, B12, C, and E, more than 20 minerals (magnesium, manganese, zinc, copper, chrome, calcium, potassium, iron), and 20 types of amino acids. Aloe extract called aloe emodin, in vials, can block the growth of cancer cells on the head and neck. Acemannan from the leaf can incite immune cells in mice to fight against cancer. In vials, di (2-ethylhexyl) phthalate (DEHP) stops the development of leukemia cells. Two studies from 2010 showed positive effect in mouse skin cancer treatment. However, in one study, some Aloe products indicated the increase of skin cancer cells. Research in Italy tested the effect of *Aloe vera* on chemotherapy treatment of persons with lung, intestine, and stomach cancer. The cancer was under control or reduced by 67% in patients who received both aloe and chemotherapy treatment, whereas by 50% with patients who only received chemotherapy. Patients using *Aloe vera* had better life quality and less side effects of chemotherapy [4–7]. Even though *Aloe vera* is generally considered as hepatoprotective [8, 9], there are also some cases described in literature where liver damage was caused by *Aloe vera* [10].

2.2 Artichoke (*Cynara scolymus*)

Artichoke is a highly appreciated plant in modern phytotherapy. The healing properties are found only in leaf but not in the flower. The most important active substances of artichoke are caffeine acid and its esters (cynarine); the concentration of which is significantly reduced in the process of drying. The other ingredients include chlorogenic acid, sesquiterpene lactones, and flavonoids. It has choleretic, antioxidative, and hepatoprotective effects. It reduces cholesterol levels in blood; it is used in dyspepsia, lack of appetite, and irritated colon; it helps in prevention of formation of cholesterol-based gallstones, and it is used in drainage treatment. Artichoke is a fairly safe plant. However, it occasionally may cause an allergic reaction. Contraindications in artichoke use include obstruction of bile ducts and artichoke allergy [11].

2.3 Cranberry (*Vaccinium macrocarpon*)

There are available data that cranberry as medicine was used as far back as among American Indians (Native American medicine). It is a bush plant with red berries originating from North America. Concentrated cranberry is called brusnicin. The most healing agent from cranberry is arbutine which acts both as antibiotic and diuretic, and it can be found in leaves. Cranberry contains hippuric acid with powerful antibacterial effect, and thus it is used in prevention or treatment of various infections (helicobacter pylori and candida). It is also recommended in treatment of urinary tract infections caused by *E. coli* [12]. Berries are rich in vitamins B and C, iron, copper, and manganese. It is highly a potent combination that strengthens weakened immune system. Berries are full of nutritious fibers that improve digestion, metabolism, and liver function. It is rich in antioxidants that reduce the harmful effect of bad blood cholesterol. It contributes to protection from free radicals and protects cardiovascular system [13]. Cranberry contains anthocyanins and proanthocyanidin which may improve eye sight and reduce blood sugar level [14]. It is a profound laxative, helps digestion, and was also very useful in prevention and treatment of gonorrhea, arthritis, rheumatism, diarrhea, skin and eye infections, sex organs, liver, cold, gallstones, prostate cancer, and urinary tract. It slows aging process and reduces underlying problems such as loss of memory and coordination. According to Canadian Journal of Microbiology, increasing concentrations of this extract reduce the bacteria's production of urease, an enzyme that contributes to the virulence of infections. Professor Nathalie Tufenkji from McGill University in Montreal states: "While the effects of cranberry in living organisms remain subject to further study, our findings highlight the role that cranberry consumption might play in the prevention of chronic infections" [15].

2.4 Beetroot (*Beta vulgaris*)

Ancient Romans were familiar with and used beetroot as food, not only its roots but its leaves as well. Although they had no idea about real reasons for its healing ability, even Dioskurides and Galen highly appreciated this vegetable and attributed great healing abilities to it. Only with the development of biochemistry it was possible to demonstrate what are the most valuable ingredients in beetroot and it is possible to confirm 2000-year-old assessment by ancient physicians. Back in 1957, researches came up with unquestionable evidence about anticancerogenic features of a beetroot. It is rich in minerals: the highest amount is potassium, then sodium, phosphorus and calcium, iron, magnesium, fluorine, also copper, sulfur, iodine, and bromine, and there are also in traces rare and valuable elements such as rubidium, cesium, and strontium. Beet's root and leaves contain apple, wine, and lemon acids. Beet also contains significant amount of cobalt used for creation of vitamin B12, B1, B2, C, and P. Amino acids (asparagine, glutamine, and betanin) are found in beetroot juice and have beneficial effect on brain and nerve activity. Betanin strengthens blood vessels, regulates blood pressure (especially in low blood pressure), reduces blood cholesterol, improves substance exchange (improves urine excretion, uric acids, and salts), as well as liver function. It increases bile excretion, and thus it is also recommended to people who have liver and bile duct diseases. It has calming effect on a nervous system; it is suitable for adrenal glands treatment; it has positive effect on stomach and intestine function, and thus it regulates feces excretion as well. This vegetable is ideal for physical and psychological strengthening of exhausted people thanks to glutamine and aspartic acids which are very important for proper brain and neural function [16, 17].

2.5 Grapefruit (*Citrus paradisi*)

Grapefruit is an evergreen tree growing up to 6 meters in height. It requires warm climate and big humidity. Fruits can grow up to 15 cm and can have yellow or orange colored peel. It is rich in vitamins C, B, P, and phytochemicals. Grapefruit strengthens immunity, regulates metabolism, and prevents cancer development, especially in lungs and colon [18]. It is abundant in minerals, magnesium, and potassium as well as organic acids, ethereal oils, sugars, microelements, pectins, and pigments. It has refreshing effect on human organism. Grapefruit also helps with atherosclerosis. Grapefruit juice has exceptional antibacterial, antifungal, and antiviral capabilities [19]. In Japan, experiments on mice showed that tumor growth stopped after mice were being injected under the skin with grapefruit extract. One grape a day is proven to reduce the risk of pancreatic cancer by half [20]. It reduces blood cholesterol levels. However, some substances found in grapefruit can have some interactions with metabolism of some drugs, if taken simultaneously, thus increasing the concentration of these drugs in blood and provoking serious, even life-threatening reactions. It is mostly connected to drugs used in treatment of cancer, depression, anxiety, angina, high blood pressure, high level of lipid cholesterol, HIV infection, different infections, and heart arrhythmias. There is evidence that even the smallest glass of grapefruit juice can cause unwanted and dangerously increased level of drugs in blood, and these effects can last for more than 3 days [21, 22].

2.6 Spirulina

Spirulina is blue-green, fresh water algae which grows in lakes and fish ponds around the world. Being 3.6-billion-year-old, it is one of the oldest residents of the planet Earth. People of Africa, North America, and Asia are using it for thousands of years. Old Aztecs consumed it in the form of dried biscuits. According to some scientists, it could solve world hunger issue since it is full of proteins, minerals, and other nutritious substances. Due to significant amount of vitamin B12, it helps in development of healthy nerve tissue and in metabolism of every cell, including those of the liver. Mineral content consists of potassium, calcium, magnesium, iron, sodium, phosphorus, zinc, and selenium. Rich in chlorophyll, it balances pH and helps in secretion of toxins out of an organism. Spirulina is the wealthiest source of beta-carotene, 10 times more than carrot. Research shows that beta-carotene is the best nutrient in fight against free radicals. Besides beta-carotene, it also contains zeaxanthin—a powerful antioxidant which has eight times stronger effect than beta-carotene [23]. Zeaxanthin has protective effect on the nervous system, brain, and eyes. Spirulina is very effective against heavy metals and medicine poisoning [24]. In case of those being overweight, it reduces hunger and cholesterol level. It protects pancreas and insulin-producing cells and thus prevents diabetes [25]. Spirulina also blocks interleukin 4 which participates in creation of allergic reaction. Studies have indicated its amazing power in stopping inflammations in the body, what is important for prevention and treatment of arthritis and many other inflammatory diseases. Due to detoxication capabilities, it was used in the Soviet Union after the Chernobyl catastrophe [26]. Having more proteins than meat, it is an excellent supplement in vegetarian and vegan diet [27].

2.7 Burdock (*Arctium lappa*)

Burdock originates from Europe and Siberia, but nowadays it can be found around the world. Burdock's root contains up to 50% of inulins, phenolic acids (caffeic and chlorogenic), and polyacetylenes. Seeds contain about 15–30% of plant oil, bitter glycoside arctiin, arctigenin, and lignans (isolappaol A and lappaol B). Burdock is traditionally used in ulcers, acne, psoriasis, and seborrhea, and it is proven to be effective in skin infections caused by gram-positive bacteria. Due to the abundance of inulins, it has beneficial effect on intestinal microflora, and it helps with regulation of the blood sugar levels. Burdock is also effective as choleretic, and it is the plant of choice for liver drainage [28]. It has anti-allergic and anti-inflammatory effects [29]. People sensitive to Asteraceae should be careful in using it because it can cause allergic reaction.

2.8 Turmeric (*Curcuma*)

Turmeric is a plant from ginger family, mostly grown in South Asia. It is a useful addition to diet and frequently subject, of clinical trials, which has numerous effects on human organism. It has anti-inflammatory effect; thus it is used in osteoarthritis and rheumatoid arthritis, ulcerous colitis, and gastritis [30]. Useful in prevention of various types of dementia and cancers, it is a powerful antioxidant and helps in healing wounds. Curcuminoids are phenolic antioxidants, and the most important representative is curcumin, found at about 3% in turmeric. Plant also contains sugars, proteins, and some fat. Despite being very biologically active even in very low concentration, the problem with curcumin is its low bioavailability. Very low amount of curcumin is absorbed in the digestive system. Therefore, new product formulas are being developed. Extracts standardized at 95% of curcumin are expanded with piperine, black pepper alkaloid, which increases curcumin absorption; liposomes with curcumin or curcumin aether oil added, that also helps with curcumin absorption. Liposomes are formulated with curcumin or curcumin aether oil added that also helps with curcumin absorption. For centuries, turmeric is used for dyspepsia problem, bloatedness, flatulence, and liver problems. Being choleretic and cholagogue, in modern phytotherapy, turmeric is recommended for difficulties with bile secretion [31]. Therefore, turmeric was an ideal plant for small gallstones problem, but the treatment must be performed under doctor's control. It has antioxidative, hepatoprotective, and antiviral effects [32]. Clinical studies confirm that it protects liver cells from hepatotoxic medicines [33]. Theoretically, there is a possibility of an interaction with coagulation medicines (acetylsalicylic acid, warfarin, heparin, and nonsteroid anti-inflammatory medicines). Extract use is not recommended during pregnancy. Hypersensitivity is possible but very rare. High dosage in sensitive people may stimulate stomach [34].

2.9 Green tea (*Camellia sinensis*)

A study in Japan compared effects of six Chinese teas on liver injuries caused by carbon tetrachloride (CCl_4) and categorized them according to their manufacturing process into green, white, yellow, oolong, black, and pu-erh. Wistar rats were given Chinese tea and afterward intraperitoneal CCl_4 or olive oil. Yellow tea significantly contributed to the protection from liver injury [35]. The difference among types of tea is related to the processing technology, time needed for the leaves to mature, or fermentation level. They have very high anticancerogenic, antioxidative, and anti-inflammatory effects. Green tea has more hepatoprotective effects compared to other types of tea, black tea, for instance. Polyphenol extract of green tea alleviated liver damage and apoptotic, oxidative, and inflammatory changes on the rat liver following hemorrhage/resuscitation [36]. In the case of mice intoxicated with iron, green tea extract reduced iron buildup in the liver, as well as creation of free radicals and oxidative stress [37]. Rats on atherogenic diet [38] or with cadmium exposure [39] had alleviated oxidative stress and liver damage thanks to green tea extract. Clinical trials indicate that consummation of green tea can reduce risk of liver disease in humans [40]. It is known that epigallocatechin gallate, the main catechin in the green tea has a modulation role in various diseases in humans, thus affecting numerous signal pathways. However, using green tea extracts can also have some unwanted effects such as hepatotoxicity, if used in concentrated form [41]. These findings confirm doubt that excessive intake of antioxidants can have adverse effect, i.e., pro-oxidative effect [42].

2.10 Dandelion (*Taraxacum officinale*)

Dandelion belongs to the family of Asteraceae. It comes from Europe and North Asia. Leaves are very tasty and a healthy addition to salads. Dandelion leaves contain a lot of minerals among which there are, in particular, potassium, beta-carotene, flavonoids, sesquiterpene lactones, taraxinic acid, and sterols. Primarily, it is used as diuretic. It has confirmed choleretic effect. Diuretic effect is significantly lower than in leaves, due to the inulin content which belongs to prebiotic fiber [43]. It has beneficial effect on intestinal microflora, and it helps with regulation of the blood sugar levels. Dandelion is used as bitter tonic for stimulating eating and in case of dyspepsia and fatty liver related to obesity [44]. It is also used in drainage cures. In case of increased cholesterol, cellulite, and weight loss, it is used as additional therapy. There is also a possibility of allergic reactions in sensitive people. It must not be used in people with bile duct obstruction. When there are gallstones, it must be taken under professional supervision. The application with digitalis and lithium preparation is not recommended. In case of gastritis and peptic ulcer, dandelion, just as all other choleretics and draining plants, should be used with caution.

2.11 Pomegranate (*Punica granatum*)

Pomegranate is one of the oldest fruit types. Rich in antioxidants, it is highly appreciated as a symbol of health, fertility, and eternal life [45]. Many studies have confirmed that it is one of the plants with the best healing effects in the world on the cardiovascular, nervous, and skeletal system. Pomegranate is an excellent source of vitamin B5, potassium, and natural phenols like ellagitannin and flavonoids. It contains phytochemicals that provoke creation of serotonin for mood improvement and estrogen for bone mass preservation, which is essential in prevention of osteoporosis. Clinical trials indicate that substances found in pomegranate, known as punicalagins, are beneficial to heart and blood veins health and have anti-inflammatory [46] and hepatoprotective effect in case of toxic liver damage. Punicalagins are also the main source of antioxidative effect. Ingredients in pomegranate inhibit growth of breast cancer, prostate cancer, colon cancer, and leukemia and prevent changes which may cause the growth of tumor [47]. It has estrogenic, anti-inflammatory, and antimicrobic properties. The research suggests that pomegranate oil protects from cancer, diabetes, obesity, and heart diseases. Being rich in antioxidants, pomegranate oil is a powerful ally in fight against aging [48].

2.12 Milk thistle (*Silybum marianum*)

Milk thistle is one of the best plants in protection and detoxication of liver. It can grow up to 2 meters in height, and it is very spiky. In many countries around the world, the plant is registered as herbal medicine. The healing part of the milk thistle is its fruit, i.e., seeds. There are numerous in vitro studies, animal studies, as well as clinical studies performed on humans. However, final conclusions regarding effects and effectiveness of this plant are still not made. What can be said with certainty is that it has hepatoprotective and hepatoregenerative effect while also increasing the level of glutathiones in liver. It does not provoke bile secretion, and thus it is appropriate for the use in cases where classic drainage plants are considered as contraindication. The plant is considered to be nontoxic and appropriate for long-term use, without pauses [49]. It is usually used for alcohol-induced liver damage, fatty liver, nonalcoholic steatohepatitis, and liver damage caused by toxins and medicines and as an auxiliary therapy for chronic hepatitis and liver cirrhosis. However, it is also very helpful in controlling blood sugar and cholesterol levels. In several minor clinical trials, milk thistle did not have any important influence on hepatitis. The treatment of patients with chronic hepatitis C resulted in reduction of serum indicators of liver damage, but without significant influence on viremia [50]. In another research, there was no significant influence on the amount of ribonucleic acid (RNA) of hepatitis C virus in the serum, on the level of ALT or the quality of life [51]. It is indicative that it can have partially protective effect as inflammatory response in hepatitis C, but it cannot play the role of antiviral agent. The possible cause of the ineffectiveness of herbal extract is probably the result of the fact that the most active components showing hepatoprotective effect are represented in much smaller percentage than if used individually. The use of silymarin resulted in the improvement of clinical symptoms of acute hepatitis, although there was no effect on inflammation process indications [52]. In a number of studies, silibinin, pharmacologically the most active flavonolignan compound in silymarin, significantly improved clinical symptoms and biochemical indications of liver function in acute and chronic hepatitis [53], alcoholic liver disease, and liver damage caused by medications [54]. Silibinin proved to be a very strong inhibitor of human liver stellate cells in vitro. They are considered to be the main producers of extracellular matrix responsible for creation of connective tissue, usually found in liver fibrosis [55]. Silymarin consists of silibinin A and B, isosilibinin A and B, silicristin, and silidianin. Plants contain about 3–6% of these compounds. There are also flavonoids, taxifolin, and quercetol. The fruit contains up to 30% of herbal oil rich in linoleic acid and phytosterols. Active ingredients found in milk thistle are not water soluble, and preparation of tea and brew makes no sense. Tinctures are also obsolete. Current extracts are factory standardized at the silymarin contents of 65–80%, and dosage is determined by the content of silymarin and not by the total volume of extract. Similar to turmeric, the problem is with the resorption of active substances from digestive system. Therefore, silymarin complex bound to lecithin was developed and thus increased its bioavailability for 5–10 times. There are very rare allergic reactions, stomach irritation, nausea, bloatedness, diarrhea, and headache. Due to the lack of data, it is not recommended to be used during pregnancy and breastfeeding. In 2013, Jinnah Postgraduate Medical Center in Karachi conducted a study aimed at the assessment of hepatoprotective role of silymarin against hepatotoxicity induced by isonicotinohydrazide. First group of rabbits was subjected to liver function test without any medicine; second group was treated with silymarin; III group received isoniazid, and IV group received combination of isoniazid and silymarin. There was no case of mortality. Group III had increased levels of bilirubin, and ALT was significantly reduced. Group IV had statistically important improvement in serum bilirubin and ALT. Hepatotoxicity induced by isonicotinohydrazide is well treated with simultaneous application of silymarin [56].

2.13 Common chicory (*Cichorii herba*)

Chicory is a wild plant that usually grows next to fields and roads. It is very popular herb in traditional medicine. Chicory root is rich in inulin and contains about 15% of sugar, some proteins, and cellulose. The most interesting compounds found in chicory are sesquiterpenic lactones, triterpenes, and flavonoids. It is used for problems with digestion, and it has hepatoprotective and anti-inflammatory effects, but also as an additional therapy in reducing high blood cholesterol values [57]. Individual compounds from the plant have proven sedative effect (lactucin and lactucopicrin). Therapeutic use is not recommended during pregnancy. It must not be used in people with bile duct obstruction. There is also a possibility of allergic reactions in sensitive people. In rare cases, there may occur nausea, diarrhea, bloatedness, and gases and use for gallstones must be under professional supervision.

2.14 Bilberry (*Vaccinium myrtillus*)

Bilberry is a deciduous shrub from Ericaceae family with the height of 20–25 cm. It is widely present in pine, spruce, and beech woods. The fruit is a round berry with 5–10 mm in diameter, dark blue colored, with thick skin and acidic-sweet taste.

Conducted research indicates the beneficial effect of blueberries on human cells in the eye retina, brain, and tumor cells [58]. Using animal model, Chinese scientists were testing the effect of blueberries on liver fibrosis. Study results indicate that blueberries can reduce degree of liver damage and the level of hyaluronic acid and ALT in blood. Based on results, authors of the study concluded that blueberries have beneficial effect on liver diseases, oxidative stress, steatosis, and even fibrosis [59].

2.15 Ubiquinone (coenzyme Q1o)

Ubiquinone belongs to the family of compounds called quinones. In 1957, it was for the first time isolated and named ubiquinone due to its wide spread in the nature. It is a substance similar to vitamins which can be found in all parts of the body and has the effect similar to that of vitamin E. However, it is probably a more powerful antioxidant than vitamin E. There are 10 known substances marked as coenzyme Qs, but coenzyme Q10 is the only one that can be found in human tissue. It has crucial role in energy production in every cell of our body. It helps circulation, stimulates immune system, increases oxygenation of tissues, and has significant antiaging effect. Human organism has the ability to synthesize Q10; however, this ability is reduced after the age of 30. The lack of Q10 is also connected to periodontal disease, diabetes, and muscular dystrophy. Belgian scientists from the University of Leuwen discovered another positive effect of coenzyme Q10, i.e., it prevents development of fatty liver related to obesity. Besides being the base for energy production, it also has series of functions with, most frequently, anti-inflammatory effect. A study in Iran indicated that Q10 as a powerful antioxidant prevents LDL from oxidation in vitro and can be a useful alternative for reduction of risk from atherosclerosis, coronary heart disease, and other health issues related to free radicals. While affecting genetic expression in liver, it reduces creation of free oxygen radicals and other “stressful” products, thus diminishing the inflammation in an organism. Q10 is an ideal partner in the fight against atherosclerosis and “fatty liver” [60]. This substance can be found in all living beings, but there are also high concentrations of it in groceries, including nut fruits and oils. There are many food additives that contain Q10.

2.16 Plant *Millettia pulchra*

It is a plant from the family of Leguminosae. It is frequently used in popular folk medicine of China, and its main ingredient is Yulangsan polysaccharide (YLSPS). Being used as a liver protection agent, it is also used as antiaging and memory-enhancing agent. The aim of the study was to search for protective effects of YLSPS against nimesulide-induced hepatotoxicity in mice. Compared to control group, YLSPS significantly reduced activities of ALT, AST, alkaline phosphatase (ALP), and bilirubin content in the serum. Antioxidative effect of YLSPS is the result of increased activity of superoxide dismutase, catalase, and glutathione peroxidase in the liver. Besides the aforementioned, the content of malondialdehyde is reduced, and histological findings were confirmed by antihepatotoxic effect as well. YLSPS showed significant inhibition of pro-inflammation mediators such as tumor necrosis alpha (TNF-α) and interleukin-6 (IL-6). Protective effect of YLSPS in nimesulide-induced liver damage can be achieved thanks to its ability to reduce oxidative stress and prevent nimesulide-induced hepatotoxicity by inhibiting critical control points of apoptosis [61].

2.17 Plant *Atalantia ceylanica*

The extract made from leaves of plant *Atalantia ceylanica* is used in a traditional medicine in Sri Lanka for a treatment of various liver diseases. Lyophilized powder of watery leaf extract was tested for its phytochemical ingredients, antioxidants, and hepatoprotective activity in vitro. Hepatotoxicity was induced in the pieces of pig's liver to test hepatoprotective activity. Parts of liver were cut off and incubated at 37°C with various concentrations of watery extract of *A. ceylanica* in the presence of ethanol during the period of 2 hours. Hepatoprotective effects are quantified through the transfer of ALT, AST, and lactate dehydrogenase (LDH) into medium [62].

2.18 Liquorice (*Glycyrrhiza glabra*)

Liquorice is a perennial and herbaceous plant from the family of legumes. It grows in the Mediterranean, close to rivers, in sandy and clay ground. The plant can grow up to 2 meters in height. The flower has specific form of Leguminosae, and the crown is yellow-white. The fruit is in the oblong pod, brown in color. Potential therapeutic effect on liver diseases is characteristic of all plants from Phyllanthus family, including *Glycyrrhizin glabra*. *Phyllanthus fraternus* indicated protective effect against dysfunctional mitochondria induced by bromobenzene in rat's liver mitochondria [63]. The extract of Phyllanthus prevented hepatotoxicity, induced by acetaminophen, by inhibiting cytochrome P459 CYP2E158. In rat's hepatocytes, phyllanthin, active ingredient, prevented intracellular growth of ROS and lipid peroxidation [64]. The extract *Phyllanthus urinaria* alleviated steatohepatitis in mice and in the culture of hepatocytes, reducing lipid buildup [65]. The extract Phyllanthus polyphyllus indicated antitumor effect in mice and human tumor cell lines MCF7 (breast cancer), HT29 colon cancer, and HepG2 (liver cancer) [66]. The lack of relevant clinical trials prevents making any conclusions on hepatoprotective effect of plants from this family. Nevertheless, rare research on patients showed that *Phyllanthus amarus* is not effective in the treatment of viral hepatitis [67], whereas glycyrrhizin a triterpenic ingredient in *Glycyrrhizin glabra* successfully reduced HCV titer in vitro [68]. In combination with interferon, glycyrrhizin showed synergic effect. Hepatoprotective effect of glycyrrhizin is related to preventing changes in cell membrane permeability. [69]. Glycyrrhetinic acid has protective effect against liver damage induced by hepatotoxic alkaloid resorcin and galactosamine [70]. In cholestatic model of liver damage, glycyrrhizin showed proaptotic effect, whereas glycyrrhetinic acid performed as powerful inhibitor of apoptosis and necrosis induced by bile acids [71]. The results of recent research indicate that glycyrrhizin prevents ischemic-reperfusional liver damage by inhibiting high-mobility group box 1 (HMGB1) early mediator of inflammation [72]. Intravenous application of Stronger Neo-Minophagen C (SNMC), a Japanese compound, containing 0.2% of glycyrrhizin, 0.1% cysteine, and 2% glycine, stopped disease progress in patients with acute seizure of autoimmune hepatitis [73]. Similarly, Korenaga et al. showed in the mice model that SNMC reduces oxidative stress and liver steatosis provoked by combination of HCV and iron [74].

2.19 Plant *Picrorhiza kurroa*

This plant is one of main forest products in Nepalese Himalaya, where it is known as Kutki. It is located far from the community, and it takes a few days walk to get to its habitat. Plant's root has long history of use in Indian Ayurvedic medicine in the digestive problem treatment. Some other uses are also suggested (asthma, liver damage, wound healing, and vitiligo); however, medical results are still not conclusive. It appears that the safe usage is based on the long history of traditional use. Kutki has hepatoprotective features. It is used for all forms of liver damage, cirrhosis, and liver inflammation. It also protects liver from damage caused by hepatitis C virus [75]. Picroliv, an iridous glycoside mixture purified from the plant, normalized indicators of acute liver damage induced by ethanol [76] and aflatoxin B1 in rats [77]. Picroliv has also effectively prevented hepatocarcinogenesis induced by N-nitrosodiethylamine, hyperlipidemia, liver steatosis, and lipid mobilization from adipose tissue in rats treated with hydrazine [78]. In rats chronically intoxicated with cadmium, picroliv alleviated pathological changes in liver and kidneys. Picroliv was also more successful at alleviating pathological changes in liver of rats intoxicated with galactosamine than its two most known ingredients picroside and kutkoside individually [79].

2.20 Barberry (*Berberis vulgaris*)

Barberry was traditionally used in the treatment of various liver diseases. Common barberry is a shrub originating from Central and Southern Europe, Northwestern Africa, and Western Asia. It grows as a deciduous bush covered in thorns and with yellow color under the bark. The fruit is a long oblong red berry and sour, containing 2–3 seeds in the inside. Berries are edible and rich in vitamin C but very sour and hard to reach because of thorns. Berberine, alkaloid isolated from plant, is one of interesting compounds which is controversial because of its toxicity in experimental animals. Thus, lethal dose in intraperitoneal application in mice was 30 mg/kg [52, 58] and 205 mg/kg in rats [54]. Research on human subjects showed good resistance, even when it is consumed in high dosages for prolonged time period. Patients with diabetes type 2 and weakened liver function managed to successfully reduce the level of glucose in blood and diminish liver damage thanks to the use of berberine without significant side effects [80]. Treatment with berberine improved liver function and alleviated signs of dyslipidemia in hyperlipidemic patients with hepatitis C and liver cirrhosis and in patients with diabetes type 2 [81]. Research conducted on 1751 dyslipidemic patients showed improvement of lipid status in blood, with significant reduction of total risk of cardiovascular diseases [82]. Just in case, berberine should be avoided during pregnancy because it can cause jaundice and fetal kernicterus [83].

2.21 Nigella (*Nigella sativa*)

Nigella and more than 20 names are related to the miraculous plant which is used for over 3000 years. It is mentioned in the Bible as black cumin. The usefulness of this plant was also described by the Prophet Mohammed s.a.w.s. in words: "Nigella contains in itself the remedy for all diseases except death." Hippocrates in his logs writes about effectiveness of this plant in healing digestive problems. In Ancient Greece, it was known as the agent for strengthening in case of physical and mental weakness of the patient. Nigella is an annual flowering plant, native to South and Southwest Asia. The fruit is a large and inflated capsule, each containing numerous seeds. Seeds are used as spice and replacement for black cumin. Seeds used for preparation of nigella oils, in large quantities, usually come from Egypt, Syria, India, Pakistan, or Ethiopia. Nigella oil is produced by so-called cold squeezing, and it is not subjected to further manipulation. What was traditionally a feature of Nigella oil, biomedicine started to confirm only since 1964. Until today, there are over 460 researches which prove its benefits for human health. The oil has beneficial effect on over 40 health conditions and more than 20 pharmacological effects. It acts as analgesic, as antibacterial [107], as anti-inflammatory, as antiulcerous, as anticholinergic, against high blood pressure, as antioxidant, as antiasthmatic, as antiviral, as bronchodilator, as antidiabetic, as hepatoprotective [84], against low blood pressure, in inulin synthesis, as antagonist to white blood cells, and as kidney protector. The oil is rich in linoleic acid, thymoquinone, nigellone, melanthin, nigellinine, damascenine, and tannin. It has been discovered that oil also contains beta-sitosterol, myristic acid, palmitic acid, stearic acid, oleic acid, linoleic acid, folic acid, and arachidonic acid. Besides the aforementioned, it is also rich in proteins; vitamins B1, B2, B6, C, and E; calcium; iron; copper; zinc; and phosphorus. Storage, squeezing, and preservation of nigella oil are very important because, in inappropriate conditions, it can have toxic effect [85].

2.22 Coumarin

Coumarin is a chemical compound found in many plants, especially in tonka seeds, woodruff, sweet grass, Perforate St John's-wort, strawberries, apricots, cherries, cinnamon, and sweet clovers. Coumarins can be found in large quantities in some oils, especially cinnamon oil, Chinese cinnamon leaf oil, and lavender oil, and in herbs like chicory, and in highest quantities in plants from the families Rutaceae and Umbelliferae [86]. There are plenty known derivatives of coumarin, synthetic or natural, and such structural diversity is the cause for many various biological activities. IMUNOMAX is dietary supplement which contains extracts of plants rich with 4-MU for liver regeneration, but it also has broad spectrum of other effects. In the world, it is considered as the strongest booster of the immune system: increases the number of T cells and the activity of NK (natural killer) cells by 300–800%, activates the immune cells (NK, LAK, and macrophage), increases cytokine production (TNF-a, gamma interferon IL-2, and IL-12), inhibits immunosuppressive cytokines like TGF-b, improves Th1/Th2 balance, and improves the function of cytotoxic white blood cells. Boosting immunity, it prevents the transition from acute into chronic form of disease, shortens disease duration, and prevents possible complications [87]. Due to immunomodulation features, there is also a possibility of its application in the treatment of chronic infectious and opportunistic infections, in brucellosis treatment [88], MRSA infections [89], for antimicrobial activity in digestive tract [90], and for antifungal activity, and some coumarins also show tuberculostatic activity. Research at the University of Texas (San Antonio) from 2005 to 2007 involving 160 patients showed that 4-MU can stop and reduce symptoms and complications of chronic virus infection with hepatitis B (HBV) and hepatitis C (HCV). This effect was noticed with naive patients, as well as with those who did not react to interferon, which was earlier used as first-line therapy for HBV and HCV infections. It is assumed that 4-MU slows down progression of hepatitis into cirrhosis and liver cancer [91]. Research into coumarin metabolism proved that rats are not suitable model for research into toxicity of coumarin for humans [92]. Coumarins generally display multiple biological activities: anticoagulative, estrogenic, photosensitive, antimicrobial, vasodilatative, antiviral against HBV and HDV [93] and HCV, and molluscicidal activity; they act as anthelmintic (in digestive system) and as sedatives and hypnotics and also indicate analgesic and hypothermal effects. Other biological activities include inhibition of aggregation of platelets, cytochrome P450 and steroid 5α-reductase, spasmolytic, choleretic [94], anticancerogenic and anti-HIV activities [95], diabetes type 1, multiple sclerosis, Alzheimer's disease, and rheumatoid arthritis. It also shows excellent effectiveness in removal of radicals, i.e., antioxidation mechanisms. Disease prevention and antioxidative features are also very important [96]. 4-MU is a powerful inhibitor of hyaluronic acid synthesis, and the result is antitumor effect; thus it can be used as chemotherapeutic agent in prostate cancer [97], breast cancer [98], stomach, melanoma, and renal cancer and prevents and helps in treatment of hepatocellular cancer [99]. Prevention and treatment of advanced prostate cancer with nontoxic agent alleviates side effects of oncological treatment, and it can also improve outcome while preserving life quality. 4-MU does not react directly with cancer itself.

It boosts immune system to be able to do its primary task—destroy tumor cells! This also explains why the compound is so effective with other types of cancer (lungs, stomach, colon, thyroid gland, ova, testes, tongue). Results are ranked from real reduction in tumor mass to stopping of growth of tumor, preventing the spread of metastases, increasing survival times, and improving of life quality during disease [100]. There are no recorded negative side effects during this therapy nor interactions with other medications. On the contrary, it is considered as an effective agent for relieving unpleasant side effects of drugs, including toxic chemotherapeutics.

3. Mechanisms of action of phytochemicals

Medicinal herbs, as a part of alternative strategy for disease prevention, which are traditionally used in folk medicine, it become important factors in human health preservation. Natural compounds with pharmacological effects for humans come into numerous interactions with internal and external cell molecules. A huge number of potential mechanisms of action of phytochemicals are suggested as a treatment for different diseases, including liver diseases. They are also independent of antioxidative activities [101]. Experiments on animals and cell cultures indicate that natural compounds can reduce pathological changes in the liver. Plants contain numerous phytochemicals: Polyphenols, phenol acids, coumarins, stilbene, tannins, lignans, and lignins [102, 103]. Polyphenols are the most famous micronutrients found in abundant amounts in diet, alongside with fruit and drinks, such as tea and red wine, as their primary source. Health effects of polyphenols depend on the amount consumed and their bioavailability. Flavonoids are the most widely spread polyphenol compounds found in plants. They can be divided into several groups: flavane, flavone, flavonol, flavanone, flavanonols, isoflavonoids, and anthocyanidins [104]. Polyphenols are proven to display a broad spectrum of pharmacological effects: Flavonoids show antiallergenic [105], anti-inflammatory, antidiabetic, cardioprotective [106], vasoprotective [107], neuroprotective [108], hepatoprotective [102], gastroprotective [109], antiviral [110], and anticancerogenic effects [111]. Flavonoids are also potential inhibitors of cellular autoimmunity [112]. Many of these compounds act as regulators of internal cellular processes such as cellular signalization or appropriate gene expression [113]. Molecular protection mechanisms and polyphenol treatment activity in different pathological conditions cannot be ascribed exclusively to their antioxidative effect but also to direct blocking of signal pathways. Anthocyanins, a type of flavonoids, for instance, affect the activity of more than 120 receptors, signal molecules, transcription factors, and genes while directly reacting with more than 20 molecular targets. Their activity depends on structure, whereas their antioxidative potential does not necessarily correlate with their ability to affect internal and external cellular processes [113].

3.1 Free radicals

Free radicals are compounds that are natural products of metabolism. Many of them have important physiological role (nitrous oxide and superoxide radical). However, increased production results in damage to the protein molecules, lipids, and genetical material. Radicals' production in an organism is incurred by numerous factors from the environment, toxic agents, polluted air, smoking, sun exposure, chronic diseases, infections, cancerogenic substances, intensive exercise, and genetic presupposition [101, 113]. Free radicals, along with other highly reactive compounds originating from oxygen, belong to the group of reactive oxygen species (ROS). ROS are result of all the processes that include the exchange of electrons, and the most frequent causes are respiratory chain in mitochondria, endoplasmic reticulum (reaction to cytochrome P 450), hemoglobin oxidation in red blood cells, special cells (leucocytes, macrophages, and others create superoxide through NADPH oxidase), and external factors (UV light, X-rays, toxic chemicals, aromatic nitrous compounds, etc.) [102].

3.2 Antioxidants

Antioxidants are a group of different compounds acting as a protection from harmful effects of free radicals. They are provided in food, like vitamins and minerals. However, many of them are produced in the organism as well. They can be of enzymatic (catalase, SOD) and nonenzymatic origin (glutathione and vitamins C and E) [102]. Free radicals are neutralized in numerous ways: By binding with pro-oxidative metal ions (iron and copper), by removing reactive compounds of oxygen (superoxide radical and hydrogen peroxide), and by inhibiting enzymes that create free radicals (NADPH oxidase). Their effects are related to slowing down aging process; reduction of cholesterol levels; reduction of risks of atherosclerosis, cardiac arrest, and stroke; prevention of creation and growth of tumors; and protection from other pathological conditions. Nowadays, various herbs and herbal preparations and medicines are more and more used in prevention and protection from liver diseases. Their most important function is antioxidative effect. Recently, significant amount of attention was dedicated to medicinal herbs with antioxidative effects [101].

4. Conclusions

Medicinal herbs, if used properly, have almost no unwanted effects, and if there are some, they are reduced to minimum. Nowadays, farming medicinal herbs without the use of artificial fertilizers and insecticides and in ecologically clean areas is preferred, in order to avoid harmful effects of pollution. Controlled picking, preservation, and processing ensure plants' health safety. Medicinal herbs are used in various pharmaceutical forms: water extracts of herbal drugs (infusions, decocts, macerates), ethanol tinctures, oil macerates, syrups, and capsules and pills. The substances important for plant's effect are very often in only one part of the plant, and thus this part in particular is used as herbal drug. Contemporary phytotherapy is a perfect combination of traditional experience and the results of modern science. Nowadays, chemical composition of the main effective substance is usually known, and the use of medicinal herbs should be rationalized and left to experts. This is particularly important when combining medicinal herbs and in using with other medicines. FDA has standards for preparation of all food supplements including medicinal herbs. FDA requires that ingredients listed on the label must actually be in the product itself, and there should be no harmful toxins, such as pesticides, for instance. FDA does not allow statements with medical indications or claims for any herbal preparation, even when its use is scientifically proven. Medicinal herbs and food supplements can have labels predicted for the category of functional food. These claims are referred to supporting body functions, for instance, that ginkgo contributes to brain health. Dietary supplements (DS) in the USA are regulated by several federal agencies whose jurisdictions overlap, Food and Drug Administration (FDA) and Federal Trade Commission (FTC), enforced by Attorney General Office (AGO) and Department of Justice (DOJ), and monitored by Center for Disease Control (CDC). FDA can remove DS from the market should there be report on unwanted event, due to contamination, misidentification, false listing, or claims and if they do not comply with Good Manufacture

Practice (GMP). FTC and AGO can enforce laws against deceiving marketing practices. Suggested improvements of existing regulatory demands are included in online DS toxic tables in a series, in order to warn in advance consumers, clinics, corporations, and governments of possible serious side effects. They can also accelerate the response rate during oversight of marketing phase IV which would enable government to have its regulatory jurisdiction [114].

Author details

Lejla Čalkić
Faculty of Medicine, University of Zenica, Zenica, Bosnia and Herzegovina

*Address all correspondence to: lejla_calkic@hotmail.com

References

[1] Negi AS, Kumar JK, Luqman S, Shanker K, Gupta MM, Khanuja SP. Recent advances in plant hepatoprotectives: A chemical and biological profile of some important leads. Medicinal Research Reviews. 2008;**28**:746-772. DOI: 10.1002/med.20115

[2] Luper S. A review of plants used in the treatment of liver disease: Part 1. Alternative Medicine Review. 1998;**3**:410-421

[3] Madrigal-Santillán E, Madrigal-Bujaidar E, Álvarez-González I, Sumaya-Martínez MT, Gutiérrez-Salinas J, et al. Review of natural products with hepatoprotective effects. World Journal of Gastroenterology. 2014;**20**(40):14787-14804. DOI: 10.3748/wjg.v20.i40.14787

[4] Nimma VL, Talla HV, Bairi JK, Gopaldas M, Bathula H, Vangdoth S. Holistic healing through herbs: Effectiveness of *Aloe vera* on post extraction socket healing. Journal of Clinical and Diagnostic Research. 2017;**11**(3):ZC83-ZC86. DOI: 10.7860/JCDR/2017/21331.9627

[5] Amjed S, Junaid K, Jafar J, Amjad T, Maqsood W, et al. Detection of antibacterial activities of Miswak, Kalonji and *Aloe vera* against oral pathogens & anti-proliferative activity against cancer cell line. BMC Complementary and Alternative Medicine. 2017;**17**(1):265. DOI: 10.1186/s12906-017-1778-0

[6] Rojas T, Bourdy G, Ruiz E, Cerapio JP, Pineau P, et al. Herbal medicine practices of patients with liver cancer in Peru. Integrative Cancer Therapies. 2018;**17**(1):52-64. DOI: 10.1177/1534735416681642

[7] Dong X, Fu J, Yin X, Yang C, Ni J. Aloe-emodin induces apoptosis in human liver HL-7702 cells through Fas death pathway and the mitochondrial pathway by generating reactive oxygen species. Phytotherapy Research. 2017;**42**(2):685-696. DOI: 10.1002/ptr.5820

[8] Cui Y, Ye Q, Wang H, Li Y, Yao W, Qian H. Hepatoprotective potential of *Aloe vera* polysaccharides against chronic alcohol-induced hepatotoxicity in mice. Journal of the Science of Food and Agriculture. 2014;**94**(9):1764-1771. DOI: 10.1002/jsfa.6489

[9] Saka WA, Akhigbe RE, Ishola OS, Ashamu EA, Olayemi OT, Adeleke GE. Hepatotherapeutic effect of *Aloe vera* in alcohol-induced hepatic damage. Pakistan Journal of Biological Sciences. 2011;**14**(14):742-746

[10] Parlati L, Voican CS, Perlemuter K, Perlemuter G. Aloe vera-induced acute liver injury: A case report and literature review. Clinics and Research in Hepatology and Gastroenterology. 2017;**41**(4):e39-e42. DOI: 10.1016/j.clinre.2016.10.002

[11] Wang M, Simon JE, Fabiola AI, He K, Zheng QY, Tadmor Y. Analysis of antioxidative phenolic compounds in artichoke (*Cynara scolymus* L.). Journal of Agricultural and Food Chemistry. 2003;**51**(3):601-608. DOI: 10.1021/jf020792b

[12] Cura Della Redazione A. Cranberry juice and urinary tract infections. Assistenza Infermieristica e Ricerca. 2016;**35**(4):206-208. DOI: 10.1702/2621.26955

[13] Baranowska M, Bartoszek A. Antioxidant and antimicrobial properties of bioactive phytochemicals from cranberry. Postępy Higieny i Medycyny Doświadczalnej (Online). 2016;**70**(0):1460-1468. DOI: 10.5604/17322693.1227896

[14] Chang CH, Chiu HF, Han YC, Chen IH, Shen YC, et al. Photoprotective effects of cranberry juice and its various fractions against blue light-induced impairment in human retinal pigment epithelial cells. Pharmaceutical Biology. 2017;**55**(1):571-580

[15] Feliciano RP, Mills CE, Istas G, Heiss C, Rodriguez-Mateos A. Absorption, metabolism and excretion of cranberry (poly)phenols in humans: A dose response study and assessment of inter-individual variability. Nutrients. 2017;**9**(3):268. DOI: 10.3390/nu9030268

[16] Hashem AN, Soliman MS, Hamed MA, Swilam NF, Lindequist U, Nawwar MA. *Beta vulgaris* subspecies cicla var. flavescens (Swiss chard): Flavonoids, hepatoprotective and hypolipidemic activities. Pharmazie. 2016;**71**(4):227-232

[17] Jain NK, Singhai AK. Protective role of *Beta vulgaris* L. leaves extract and fractions on ethanol-mediated hepatic toxicity. Acta Poloniae Pharmaceutica. 2012;**69**(5):945-950

[18] Mandadi KK, Jayaprakasha GK, Bhat NG, Patil BS. Red Mexican grapefruit: A novel source for bioactive limonoids and their antioxidant activity. Zeitschrift für Naturforschung. Section C. 2007;**62**(3-4):179-188

[19] Shailender J, Ravi PR, Saha P, Myneni S. Oral pharmacokinetic interaction of ester rich fruit juices and pharmaceutical excipients with tenofovir disoproxil fumarate in male Wistar rats. Xenobiotica 2017;**47**(12):1104-1111. DOI: 10.1080/00498254.2016.1269375

[20] Cholewka-Stafińska M, Polaniak R, Kardas M, Grajek M, Grochowska-Niedworok E. Interaction of oral form anticancer drugs with grapefruit juice. Polski Merkuriusz Lekarski. 2017;**42**(247):30-33

[21] Onakpoya I, O'Sullivan J, Heneghan C, Thompson M. The effect of grapefruits (*Citrus paradisi*) on body weight and cardiovascular risk factors: A systematic review and meta-analysis of randomized clinical trials. Critical Reviews in Food Science and Nutrition. 2017;**57**(3):602-612. DOI: 10.1080/10408398.2014.901292

[22] Bailey DG. Predicting clinical relevance of grapefruit—Drug interactions: A complicated process. Journal of Clinical Pharmacy and Therapeutics. 2017;**42**(2):125-127. DOI: 10.1111/jcpt.12463

[23] Aissaoui O, Amiali M, Bouzid N, Belkacemi K, Bitam A. Effect of *Spirulina platensis* ingestion on the abnormal biochemical and oxidative stress parameters in the pancreas and liver of alloxan-induced diabetic rats. Pharmaceutical Biology. 2017;**55**(1):1304-1312. DOI: 10.1080/13880209.2017.1300820

[24] Peter SJ, Basha SK, Giridharan R, Lavinya BU, Sabina EP. Suppressive effect of *Spirulina fusiformis* on diclofenac-induced hepato-renal injury and gastrointestinal ulcer in Wistar albino rats: A biochemical and histological approach. Biomedicine & Pharmacotherapy. 2017;**88**:11-18. DOI: 10.1016/j.biopha.2017.01.032

[25] Gargouri M, Magné C, El Feki A. Hyperglycemia, oxidative stress, liver damage and dysfunction in alloxan-induced diabetic rat are prevented by Spirulina supplementation. Nutrition Research. 2016;**36**(11):1255-1268. DOI: 10.1016/j.nutres.2016.09.011

[26] Cheng J, Lu H, He X, Yang W, Zhou J, Cen K. Mutation of Spirulina sp. by nuclear irradiation to improve growth rate under 15% carbon dioxide in flue gas. Bioresource Technology. 2017;**238**:650-656. DOI: 10.1016/j.biortech.2017.04.107

[27] Vázquez-Velasco M, González-Torres L, García-Fernández RA, Méndez MT, Bastida S, et al. Glucomannan or Glucomannan plus Spirulina-enriched squid-Surimi diets reduce histological damage to liver and heart in Zucker fa/fa rats fed a cholesterol-enriched and non-cholesterol-enriched Atherogenic diet. Journal of Medicinal Food. 2017;**20**(6):618-625. DOI: 10.1089/jmf.2016.0157

[28] De Souza PF, da Silva Diamante MA, Foglio MA, Camargo Cde A, Aoyama H, et al. Hepatoprotective effect of *Arctium lappa* root extract on cadmium toxicity in adult Wistar rats. Biological Trace Element Research. 2014;**160**(2):250-257. DOI: 10.1007/s12011-014-0040-6

[29] Sohn EH, Jang SA, Joo H, Park S, Kang SC, Lee CH, et al. Anti-allergic and anti-inflammatory effects of butanol extract from *Arctium lappa* L. Clinical and Molecular Allergy. 2011;**9**(1):4. DOI: 10.1186/1476-7961-9-4

[30] Yiu WF, Kwan PL, Wong CY, Kam TS, Chiu SM, Chan SW, et al. Attenuation of fatty liver and prevention of hypercholesterolemia by extract of *Curcuma longa* through regulating the expression of CYP7A1, LDL-receptor, HO-1, and HMG-CoA reductase. Journal of Food Science. 2011;**76**:H80-H89. DOI: 10.1111/j.1750-3841.2011.02042.x

[31] El-Shahat M, El-Abd S, Alkafafy M,El-Khatib G. Potential chemoprevention of diethylnitrosamine-induced hepatocarcinogenesis in rats: Myrrh (Commiphora molmol) vs. turmeric (Curcuma longa). Acta Histochemica. 2012;**114**(5):421-428. DOI: 10.1016/j.acthis.2011.08.002

[32] Kim HJ, Yoo HS, Kim JC, Park CS, Choi MS, Kim M, et al. Antiviral effect of *Curcuma longa* Linn extract against hepatitis B virus replication. Journal of Ethnopharmacology. 2009;**124**:189-196. DOI: 10.1016/j.jep.2009.04.046

[33] Zhang A, Li Q, On X, Si D, Liu C. Interactions between transporters and herbal medicines/drugs: A focus on hepatoprotective compounds. Current Drug Metabolism. 2015;**16**(10):911-918

[34] Li Q, Zhang M, Zhou X, Wang S, Shu G, Yang W. Effect of different semial rhizomes on yield and quality of *Curcuma longa*. Zhongguo Zhong Yao Za Zhi. 2009;**34**(5):542-543

[35] Hashimoto T, Goto M, Sakakibara H, Oi N, Okamoto M, Kanazawa K. Yellow tea is more potent than other types of tea in suppressing liver toxicity induced by carbon te-trachloride in rats. Phytotherapy Research. 2007;**21**:668-670. DOI: 10.1002/ptr.2132

[36] Saewong T, Ounjaijean S, Mundee Y, Pattanapanyasat K, Fucharoen S, Porter JB, et al. Effects of green tea on iron accumulation and oxidative stress in livers of iron-challenged thalassemic mice. Medicinal Chemistry. 2010;**6**:57-64

[37] Ramesh E, Jayakumar T, Elanchezhian R, Sakthivel M, Geraldine P, Thomas PA. Green tea catechins, alleviate hepatic lipidemic-oxidative injury in Wistar rats fed an atherogenic diet. Chemico-Biological Interactions. 2009;**180**:10-19. DOI: 10.1016/j.cbi.2009.02.013

[38] Hamden K, Carreau S, Marki FA, Masmoudi H, El Feki A. Positive effects of green tea on hepatic dysfunction, lipid peroxidation and antioxidant defence depletion induced by cadmium. Biological Research. 2008;**41**:331-339. DOI: S0716-97602008000300009

[39] Jin X, Zheng RH, Li YM. Green tea consumption and liver disease: A systematic review. Liver International. 2008;**28**:990-996. DOI: 10.1111/j.1478-3231.2008.01776.x

[40] Molinari M, Watt KD, Kruszyna T, Nelson R, Walsh M, Huang WY, et al. Acute liver failure induced by green tea extracts: Case report and review of the literature. Liver Transplantation. 2006;**12**:1892-1895

[41] Verhelst X, Burvenich P, Van Sassenbroeck D, Gabriel C, Lootens M, Baert D. Acute hepatitis after treatment for hair loss with oral green tea extracts (*Camellia sinensis*). Acta Gastroenterologica Belgica. 2009;**72**:262-264

[42] Clare BA, Conroy RS, Spelman K. The diuretic effect in human subjects of an extract of *Taraxacum officinale folium* over a single day. Journal of Alternative and Complementary Medicine. 2009;**15**(8):929-934. DOI: 10.1089/acm.2008.0152

[43] Davaatseren M, Hur HJ, Yang HJ, Hwang JT, Park JH, Kim HJ, et al. Taraxacum official (dandelion) leaf extract alleviates high-fat diet-induced nonalcoholic fatty liver. Food and Chemical Toxicology. 2013;**58**:30-36. DOI: 10.1016/j.fct.2013.04.023

[44] Dassprakash MV, Arun R, Abraham SK, Premkumar K. In vitro and in vivo evaluation of antioxidant and antigenotoxic potential of *Punica granatum* leaf extract. Pharmaceutical Biology. 2012;**50**(12):1523-1530. DOI: 10.3109/13880209.2012.689771

[45] Costantini S, Rusolo F, De Vito V, Moccia S, Picariello G, Capone F, et al. Potential anti-inflammatory effects of the hydrophilic fraction of pomegranate (*Punica granatum* L.) seed oil on breast cancer cell lines. Molecules. 2014;**19**(6):8644-8660. DOI: 10.3390/molecules19068644

[46] Shaban NZ, El-Kersh MA, Bader-Eldin MM, Kato SA, Hamoda AF. Effect of *Punica granatum* (pomegranate) juice extract on healthy liver and hepatotoxicity induced by diethylnitrosamine and phenobarbital in male rats. Journal of Medicinal Food. 2014;**17**(3):339-349. DOI: 10.1089/jmf.2012.0306

[47] Zou X, Yan C, Shi Y, Cao K, Xu J, Wang X, et al. Mitochondrial dysfunction in obesity-associated nonalcoholic fatty liver disease: The protective effects of pomegranate with its active component punicalagin. Antioxidants & Redox Signaling. 2014;**21**(11):1557-1570. DOI: 10.1089/ars.2013.5538

[48] Hiraganahalli BD, Chinampudur VC, Dethe S, Mundkinajeddu D, Pandre MK, Balachandran J, et al. Hepatoprotective and antioxidant activity of standardized herbal extracts. Pharmacognosy Magazine. 2012;**8**(30):116-123. DOI: 10.4103/0973-1296.96553

[49] Pradhan SC, Girish C. Hepatoprotective herbal drug, silymarin from experimental pharmacology to clinical medicine. The Indian Journal of Medical Research. 2006;**124**:491-504

[50] Torres M, Rodríguez-Serrano F, Rosario DJ, Rodríguez-Perez F, Toro DH. Does Silybum marianum play a role in the treatment of chronic hepatitis C? Puerto Rico Health Sciences Journal. 2004;**23**(2 Suppl):69-74. PMID: 16929590

[51] Gordon A, Hobbs DA, Bowden DS, Bailey MJ, Mitchell J, Francis AJ, et al. Effects of *Silybum marianum* on serum hepatitis C virus RNA, alanine aminotransferase levels and well-being in patients with chronic hepatitis C. Journal of Gastroenterology and Hepatology. 2006;**21**:275-280

[52] El-Kamary SS, Shardell MD, Abdel-Hamid M, Ismail S, El-Ateek M, Metwally M, et al. A randomized controlled trial to assess the safety and

efficacy of silymarin on symptoms, signs and biomarkers of acute hepatitis. Phytomedicine. 2009;**16**:391-400

[53] Ahmed-Belkacem A, Ahnou N, Barbotte L, Wychowski C, Pallier C, Brillet R, et al. Silibinin and related compounds are direct inhibitors of hepatitis C virus RNA-dependent RNA polymerase. Gastroenterology. 2010;**138**:1112-1122

[54] Ferenci P, Scherzer TM, Kerschner H, Rutter K, Beinhardt S, Hofer H, et al. Silibinin is a potent antiviral agent in patients with chronic hepatitis C not responding to pegylated interferon/ribavirin therapy. Gastroenterology. 2008;**135**:1561-1567

[55] Falasca K, Ucciferri C, Mancino P, Vitacolonna E, De Tullio D, Pizzigallo E, et al. Treatment with silybin-vitamin E-phospholipid complex in patients with hepatitis C infection. Journal of Medical Virology. 2008;**80**:1900-1906. DOI: 10.1002/jmv.21292

[56] Jahan S, Khan M, Imran S, Sair M. The hepatoprotective role of Silymarin in isoniazid induced liver damage of rabbits. The Journal of the Pakistan Medical Association. 2015;**65**(6):620-622

[57] Li H, Liu XQ, Zhang B, Ni L, Ling ZJ. Effects of active component in Cichorii on lipid metabolism of rat with hypertriglyceridemia complicated by hyperuricemia and hyperglycemia. Zhong Xi Yi Jie He Xue Bao. 2008;**6**(2):57-62

[58] Domitrović R, Jakovac H. Effects of standardized bilberry fruit extract (Mirtoselect®) on resolution of CCl_4-induced liver fibrosis in mice. Food and Chemical Toxicology. 2011;**49**(4):848-854. DOI: 10.1016/j.fct.2010.12.006

[59] Tang X, Shen T, Jiang X, Xia M, Sun X, Guo H, et al. Purified anthocyanins from bilberry and black currant attenuate hepatic mitochondrial dysfunction and steatohepatitis in mice with methionine and choline deficiency. Journal of Agricultural and Food Chemistry. 2015;**63**(2):552-561. DOI: 10.1021/jf504926n

[60] Ahmadvand H, Mabuchi H, Nohara A, Kobayahi J, Kawashiri MA. Effects of coenzyme Q (10) on LDL oxidation in vitro. Acta Medica Iranica. 2013;**51**(1):12-18

[61] Nguyen V, Huang J, Doan V, Lin X, Tang X, Huang Y, et al. Hepatoprotective effects of Yulangsan polysaccharide against nimesulide-induced liver injury in mice. Journal of Ethnopharmacology. 2015;**172**:273-280. DOI: 10.1016/j.jep.2015.06.048

[62] Fernando CD, Soysa P. Total phenolic, flavonoid contents, in-vitro antioxidant activities and hepatoprotective effect of aqueous leaf extract of *Atalantia ceylanica*. BMC Complementary and Alternative Medicine. 2014;**14**:395. DOI: 10.1186/1472-6882-14-395

[63] Gopi S, Setty OH. Protective effect of *Phyllanthus fraternus* against bromobenzene induced mitochondrial dysfunction in rat liver mitochondria. Food and Chemical Toxicology. 2010;**48**:2170-2175

[64] Chirdchupunseree H, Pramyothin P. Protective activity of phyllanthin in ethanol-treated primary culture of rat hepatocytes. Journal of Ethnopharmacology. 2010;**128**:172-176. DOI: 10.1016/j.jep.2010.01.003

[65] Shen B, Yu J, Wang S, Chu ES, Wong VW, Zhou X, et al. *Phyllanthus urinaria* ameliorates the severity of nutritional steatohepatitis both in vitro and in vivo. Hepatology. 2008;**47**:473-483

[66] Koike K. Expression of junB is markedly stimulated by glycyrrhizin in a human hepatoma cell line. Oncology Reports. 2011;**25**:609-617. DOI: 10.3892/or.2011.1137

[67] Xia Y, Luo H, Liu JP, Gluud C. Phyllanthus species for chronic hepatitis B virus infection. Cochrane Database of Systematic Reviews. 2011;**4**:CD008960

[68] Ashfaq UA, Masoud MS, Nawaz Z, Riazuddin S. Glycyrrhizin as antiviral agent against hepatitis C virus. Journal of Translational Medicine. 2011;**9**:112. DOI: 10.1186/1479-5876-9-112

[69] Nakamura T, Fujii T, Ichihara A. Enzyme leakage due to change of membrane permeability of primary cultured rat hepatocytes treated with various hepatotoxins and its prevention by glycyrrhizin. Cell Biology and Toxicology. 1985;**1**:285-295

[70] Lin G, Nnane IP, Cheng TV. The effects of pretreatment with glycyrrhizin and glycyrrhetinic acid on the retrorsine-induced hepatotoxicity in rats. Toxicon. 1999;**37**:1259-1270

[71] Gumpricht E, Dahl R, Devereaux MW, Sokol RJ. Licorice compounds glycyrrhizin and 18β-glycyrrhetinic acid are potent modulators of bile acid-induced cytotoxicity in rat hepatocytes. The Journal of Biological Chemistry. 2005;**280**:10556-10563. DOI: 10.1074/jbc.M411673200

[72] Ogiku M, Kono H, Hara M, Tsuchiya M, Fujii H. Glycyrrhizin prevents liver injury by inhibition of high-mobility group box 1 production by kupffer cells after ischemia-reperfusion in rats. The Journal of Pharmacology and Experimental Therapeutics. 2011;**339**(1):93-98. DOI: 10.1124/jpet.111.182592

[73] Yasui S, Fujiwara K, Tawada A, Fukuda Y, Nakano M, Yokosuka O. Efficacy of intravenous glycyrrhizin in the early stage of acute onset autoimmune hepatitis. Digestive Diseases and Sciences. 2011. (In press)

[74] Korenaga M, Hidaka I, Nishina S, Sakai A, Shinozaki A, Gondo T, et al. A glycyrrhizin-containing preparation reduces hepatic steatosis induced by hepatitis C virus protein and iron in mice. Liver International. 2011;**31**:552-560

[75] Girish C, Pradhan SC. Drug development for liver diseases: Focus on picroliv, ellagic acid and curcumin. Fundamental & Clinical Pharmacology. 2008;**22**:623-632. DOI: 10.1111/j.1472-8206.2008.00618.x

[76] Saraswat B, Visen PK, Patnaik GK, Dhawan BN. Ex vivo and in vivo investigations of picroliv from *Picrorhiza kurroa* in an alcohol intoxication model in rats. Journal of Ethnopharmacology. 1999;**66**:263-269

[77] Rastogi R, Srivastava AK, Rastogi AK. Biochemical changes induced in liver and serum of aflatoxin B1-treated male wistar rats: Preventive effect of picroliv. Pharmacology & Toxicology. 2001;**88**:53-58

[78] Vivekanandan P, Gobianand K, Priya S, Vijayalakshmi P, Karthikeyan S. Protective effect of picroliv against hydrazine-induced hyperlipidemia and hepatic steatosis in rats. Drug and Chemical Toxicology. 2007;**30**:241-252

[79] Lee HS, Li L, Kim HK, Bilehal D, Li W, Lee DS, et al. The protective effects of *Curcuma longa* Linn. extract on carbon tetrachloride-induced hepatotoxicity in rats via upregulation of Nrf2. Journal of Microbiology and Biotechnology. 2010;**20**:1331-1338

[80] Zhang H, Wei J, Xue R, Wu JD, Zhao W, Wang ZZ, et al. Berberine lowers blood glucose in type 2 diabetes mellitus patients through increasing insulin receptor expression. Metabolism. 2010;**59**(2):285-292. DOI: 10.1016/j.metabol.2009.07.029

[81] Gu Y, Zhang Y, Shi X, Li X, Hong J, Chen J, et al. Effect of traditional Chinese medicine

berberine on type 2 diabetes based on comprehensive metabonomics. Talanta. 2010;**81**:766-772

[82] Trimarco B, Benvenuti C, Rozza F, Cimmino CS, Giudice R, Crispo S. Clinical evidence of efficacy of red yeast rice and berberine in a large controlled study versus diet. Mediterranean Journal of Nutrition and Metabolism. 2011;**4**:133-139

[83] Ashraf S, Anjum AA, Ahmad A, Firyal S, Sana S, Latif AA. In vitro activity of *Nigella sativa* against antibiotic resistant Salmonella enterica. Environmental Toxicology and Pharmacology. 2017;**58**:54-58. DOI: 10.1016/j.etap.2017.12.017

[84] Omar NM, Mohammed MA. The impact of black seed oil on tramadol-induced hepatotoxicity: Immunohistochemical and ultrastructural study. Acta Histochemica. 2017;**119**(5):543-554

[85] Arslan BA, Isik FB, Gur H, Ozen F, Catal T. Apoptotic effect of *Nigella sativa* on human lymphoma U937 cells. Pharmacognosy Magazine. 2017;**13**(3):S628-S632. DOI: 10.4103/pm.pm_93_17

[86] Molnar M, Čačić M. Biološka aktivnost derivata kumarina—Pregledni rad. Croatian Journal of Food Science and Technology. 2011;**3**(2):55-64

[87] Lacy A, O'Kennedy R. Studies on coumarins and coumarin-related compounds to determine their therapeutic role in the treatment of cancer. Current Pharmaceutical Design. 2004;**10**(30):3797-3811

[88] Shi Y, Zhou CH. Synthesis and evaluation of a class of new coumarin triazole derivatives as potential antimicrobial agents. Bioorganic & Medicinal Chemistry Letters. 2011;**21**:956-960

[89] Zuo GY, Wang CJ, Han J, Li YQ, Wang GC. Synergism of coumarins from the Chinese drug *Zanthoxylum nitidum* with antibacterial agents against methicillin-resistant *Staphylococcus aureus* (MRSA). Phytomedicine. 2016;**23**(14):1814-1820. DOI: 10.1016/j.phymed.2016.11.001

[90] Fang Y, Wang H, Zhu W, Wang L, Liu H, Xu X, et al. Antioxidative properties of 4-methylumbelliferone are related to antibacterial activity in the silkworm (*Bombyx mori*) digestive tract. Journal of Comparative Physiology. B. 2014;**184**(6):699-708. DOI: 10.1007/s00360-014-0840-1

[91] Hoyumpa AM, Leach CT, Pavlin D. University of Texas Health Science. 4-Methylumbelliferone as a treatment for chronic HBV/HCV. (https://clinicaltrials.gov/ct2/show/NCT00225537)

[92] Kaneko M, Futamura Y, Tsukuda S, Kondoh Y, Sekine T, Hirano H, et al. Chemical array system, a platform to identify novel hepatitis B virus entry inhibitors targeting sodium taurocholate cotransporting polypeptide. Scientific Reports. 2018;**8**(1):2769. DOI: 10.1038/s41598-018-20987-w

[93] Tsay SC, Lin SY, Huang WC, Hsu MH, Hwang KC, Lin CC, et al. Synthesis and structure-activity relationships of imidazole-coumarin conjugates against hepatitis C virus. Molecules. 2016;**21**(2):228. DOI: 10.3390/molecules21020228

[94] Zhou P, Takaishi Y, Duan H, Chen B, Honda G, Itoh M, et al. Coumarins and bicoumarin from Ferula sumbul: Anti-HIV activity and inhibition of cytokinerelease. Phytochemistry. 2000;**53**:689-697

[95] Nagy N, Kuipers HF, Marshall PL, Wang E, Kaber G, Bollyky PL. Hyaluronan in immune dysregulation

and autoimmune diseases. Matrix Biology. 2018;67. pii: S0945-053X(17)30440-7. DOI: 10.1016/j.matbio.2018.03.022

[96] Al-Majedy YK, Al-Amiery AA, Kadhum AA, Mohamad AB. Antioxidant activities of 4-methylumbelliferone derivatives. PLoS One. 2016;**11**(5):e0156625. DOI: 10.1371/journal.pone.0156625. eCollection 2016

[97] Cheng XB, Sato N, Kohi S, Koga A, Hirata K. 4-Methylumbelliferone inhibits enhanced hyaluronan synthesis and cell migration in pancreatic cancer cells in response to tumor-stromal interactions. Oncology Letters. 2018;**15**(5):6297-6301. DOI: 10.3892/ol.2018.8147

[98] Karalis TT, Heldin P, Vynios DH, Neill T, Buraschi S, Iozzo RV, et al. Tumor-suppressive functions of 4-MU on breast cancer cells of different ER status: Regulation of hyaluronan/HAS2/CD44 and specific matrix effectors. Matrix Biology. 2018;67. DOI: 10.1016/j.matbio.2018.04.007

[99] Piccioni F, Fiore E, Bayo J, Atorrasagasti C, Peixoto E, Rizzo M, et al. 4-methylumbelliferone inhibits hepatocellular carcinoma growth by decreasing IL-6 production and angiogenesis. Glycobiology. 2015;**25**(8):825-835. DOI: 10.1093/glycob/cwv023

[100] Travis JY, Luis EL, Soum DL, Nicolas O, Georgios K, Andre J, et al. Dietary supplement 4-methylumbelliferone: An effective chemopreventive and therapeutic agent for prostate cancer. Journal of the National Cancer Institute. 2015;**107**(7):1. DOI: 10.1093/jnci/djv085

[101] Domitrović R. Hepatoprotektivno djelovanje fitokemikalija. Medicina Fluminensis. 2012;**48**(1):4-14

[102] Domitrović R, Jakovac H, Tomac J, Šain I. Liver fibrosis in mice induced by carbon tetrachloride and its reversion by luteolin. Toxicology and Applied Pharmacology. 2009;**241**:311-321. DOI: 10.1016/j.taap.2009.09.001

[103] Naczk M, Shahidi F. Phenolics in cereals, fruits and vegetables: Occurrence, extraction and analysis. Journal of Pharmaceutical and Biomedical Analysis. 2006;**41**:1523-1542. DOI: 10.1016/j.jpba.2006.04.002

[104] Burda S, Oleszek W. Antioxidant and antiradical activities of flavonoids. Journal of Agricultural and Food Chemistry. 2001;**49**(6):2774-2779

[105] Kawai M, Hirano T, Higa S, Arimitsu J, Maruta M, Kuwahara Y, et al. Flavonoids and related compounds as anti-allergic substances. Allergology International. 2007;**56**:113-123. DOI: 10.2332/allergolint.R-06-135

[106] Cook NC, Samman S. Flavonoid-schemistry, metabolism, cardioprotective effects, and dietary sources. The Journal of Nutritional Biochemistry. 1996;7:66-76

[107] Bell DR, Gochenaur K. Direct vasoactive and vasoprotective properties of anthocyanin-rich extracts. Journal of Applied Physiology. 2006;**100**:1164-1170. DOI: 10.1152/japplphysiol.00626.2005

[108] Schroeter H, Williams RJ, Matin R, Iversen L, Rice-Evans CA. Phenolic antioxidants attenuate neuronal cell death following uptake of oxidized low-density lipoprotein. Free Radical Biology & Medicine. 2000;**29**:1222-1233

[109] Zayachkivska OS, Konturek SJ, Drozdowicz D, Konturek PC, Brzozowski T, Ghegotsky MR. Gastroprotective effects of flavonoids in plant extracts. Journal of Physiology and Pharmacology. 2005;**56**(1 Suppl):219-231

[110] Wei F, Ma SC, Ma LY, But PP, Lin RC, Khan IA. Antiviral flavonoids from the seeds of *Aesculus chinensis*. Journal of Natural Products. 2004;**67**:650-653. DOI: 10.1021/np030470h

[111] Seelinger G, Merfort I, Wölfle U, Schempp CM. Anti-carcinogenic effects of the flavonoid luteolin. Molecules. 2008;**13**:2628-2651

[112] Verbeek R, Plomp AC, van Tol EA, van Noort JM. The flavones luteolin and apigenin inhibit in vitro antigen-specific proliferation and interferon-gamma production by murine and human autoimmune T cells. Biochemical Pharmacology. 2004;**68**:621-629. DOI: 10.1016/j.bcp.2004.05.012

[113] Domitrović R. The molecular basis for the pharmacological activity of anthocyans. Current Medicinal Chemistry. 2011;**18**:4454-4469

[114] Brown AC. An overview of herb and dietary supplement efficacy, safety and government regulations in the United States with suggested improvements. Part 1 of 5 series. Food and Chemical Toxicology. 2017;**107**(Pt A):449-471. DOI: 1016/j.fct.2016.11.001

Chapter 6

Molecular and Cellular Aspects of Cirrhosis and How an Adenosine Derivative Could Revert Fibrosis

Jesús Rafael Rodríguez-Aguilera,
Rebeca Pérez-Cabeza de Vaca, Nuria Guerrero-Celis,
Gabriela Velasco-Loyden, Mariana Domínguez-López,
Félix Recillas-Targa and Victoria Chagoya de Sánchez

Abstract

Hepatic fibrosis occurs in response to persistent liver damage and is characterized by an excessive accumulation of extracellular matrix. When the damage is prolonged, there is a chronic inflammation and persistent hepatic fibrosis eventually leads to cirrhosis, where in addition to the scar, there is an important vascular remodeling associated with portal hypertension and, if decompensated, leads to death or can develop hepatocellular carcinoma. We have been studying the pharmacologic functions of adenosine, finding that a derivative of this nucleoside, IFC-305, shows hepatoprotective effects in a CCl_4-induced rat cirrhosis model where it reverses liver fibrosis through modulation of fibrosis-related genes and by ameliorating hepatic function. Furthermore, this compound has the property to rescue cell cycle inhibition *in vivo*, prevents hepatic stellate cell activation, modulates anti-inflammatory macrophage polarization, and favors a chromatin context that could decrease the genomic instability and characteristics of cirrhosis, enabling the recovery of gene expression profile. Here we show results that contribute to the comprehension of molecular and cellular mechanism of cirrhosis, give the opportunity to suggest biomarkers to the early diagnostic of this pathology, and constitute the fundaments to suggest IFC-305 as a coadjuvant for treatment of this disease.

Keywords: liver fibrosis reversion, adenosine, Kupffer cells, hepatic stellate cells, cell cycle, epigenetics

1. Introduction

Cirrhosis is the 14th dead cause worldwide in adults [1]; this pathology represents an hepatocellular alteration, which is defined histologically by a vascular remodeling that triggers formation of fibrotic interconnected septum that wraps the entire liver tissue and divides the parenchyma in nodules [2]; as a consequence, there is a reduction in hepatocellular mass as well as liver function and blood flow alterations. These pathologic characteristics are independent of disease etiology, which mainly could be alcoholic, biliary, and directed by viral or chronic hepatitis [3].

In the past, cirrhosis was considered as an irreversible illness, but there is evidence, which suggests that when there is an arrest of the viral or nonviral mayor cirrhotic-generator insult, it is possible to resolve fibrosis [4–9]. This is evident in successfully chronic hepatitis C treatment, in fibrosis resolution in hemochromatosis patients with effective treatment, and also in alcoholic liver illness patient who has suspended alcohol consumption [10]. A group of histopathological injuries of “reverted cirrhosis” has been described in the “hepatic reparatory complex” [9] including a thin, incomplete and perforated septum, through which hepatocytes are evident; there is a hepatocyte growing in terminal hepatic venules and little cumulus of thick collagen fibers in the parenchymal sinusoids [2]. Nevertheless, this disease could be considered as a pre-neoplastic state considering that 80% of hepatocellular carcinoma originated from cirrhosis [11].

This pathology is a silence one; generally it courses without symptoms, whereby its development confers a significant morbidity and mortality risk, and progression to this terminal state of chronic liver injury is slow, around 20–40 years [12]. Thanks to advances in the understanding of chromatin organization and rapid progress in sequencing technology, it has been clear that not only genetics but also epigenetics influence both normal human biology and diseases [13]; the combinatorial of these both factors could influence on speed of disease development, generating changes in chromatin, an inflammatory process and hepatic stellate cell (HSC) activation, triggering a pro-fibrotic environment and if it is perpetuated, the cirrhosis establishment. In this section, we will get deep into molecular and cellular aspects of cirrhosis and how an adenosine derivative could reverse this pathology through generating an anti-inflammatory environment and blocking HSC activation, modulating cell cycle and mediating epigenetic changes which reduce altered expressed genes.

2. Biochemical and physiological alteration of liver during cirrhosis and hepatoprotective effects of an adenosine derivative

Cirrhosis has a complex cellular and molecular dynamic that should be approached using laboratory models that could be animal or cell cultures. One of the most studied cirrhotic models employs carbon tetrachloride (CCl_4) to generate the pathology. This compound is a hepatic and renal toxic, whose effect is produced by two different mechanisms: the first one is related with the alteration of hepatocyte capacity to bind triacylglycerides to transporter lipoproteins, triggering an intracellular lipid accumulation and fatty degeneration of the liver; the second mechanism consists in the formation of metabolites extremely toxic, which lead to cell death and centrilobular hepatic necrosis [14]. This toxic compound is a substrate of P450 cytochrome that transforms it into $CCl_3\cdot$ radicals, and these radicals generate $CCl_3OO\cdot$ when it reacts with molecular oxygen. Since $CCl_3\cdot$ radicals react with cell membranes inducing lipid peroxidation, it has been proposed that the main cause of hepatic illness by CCl_4 is the membrane damage by the free radical chain reaction, and probably, the initial event is related with mitochondrion membrane damage [15]. Nevertheless, it is important to say that this model, unlike what happens in the human, progresses to hepatocellular carcinoma with low frequency, so that it permits only the evaluation of cirrhotic state.

Rats are intraperitoneal treated with 0.04 g/kg body weight of CCl_4 three times per week, during 10 weeks. After this time it is possible to observe a liver distortion, the formation of nodules, bilirubin accumulation and hepatomegaly [16], the generation of a fibrotic area of 16% of the tissue, and a reduction in parenchyma surface to around 78%. As a consequence of these liver architecture changes, there are alterations of liver function: serum samples of cirrhotic rats display elevated AST,

ALT, and bilirubin levels and albumin are relatively reduced [17]. Furthermore, there is a reduction in ATP level with slow recovery after 5 weeks with saline. All of these altered parameters reflect chronic hepato-biliary injury.

Since 1967, our laboratory has been studying the pharmacologic effects of adenosine on hepatic metabolism [18], finding that this nucleoside increases hepatocyte energetic charge [19], an effect which is able to increase metabolic fluxes [20]; it increases glycogen synthesis, blocks fatty acid oxidation [21], and maintains cell redox state. Some of the pharmacologic effects of adenosine on hepatotoxicity are: prevention of fatty liver disease [21], recovery of basal energetic state which was reduced by toxic agents [22], maintenance of redox balance between cytosol and mitochondrion [23], prevention of CCl_4-induced necrosis [24], avoiding free radical propagation during CCl_4 metabolism [25], and modulation of the blood flux of hepatic artery [23]. Furthermore, adenosine is able to reduce 50% collagen accumulation in a cirrhosis prevention model, thanks to the increase of liver collagenolytic activity hand by hand with an improvement of liver function [26–31]. These findings allowed us to propose adenosine as possible treatment to reverse cirrhosis.

In order to understand the mechanism of action of adenosine, we generated several derivatives and compared their hepatoprotective properties against adenosine, because this nucleoside is subject of an active metabolism within the cell resulting in a short half-life of the nucleoside but with capability of metabolic modulation; it could be phosphorylated by adenosine kinase, deaminated to inosine by adenosine deaminase, or transformed to S-adenosylhomocysteine by S-adenosylhomocysteine hydrolase [32].We found that aspartic salt of this nucleoside, now denominated IFC-305, presents a better protection against lethal dose of CCl_4 using a fourth of the dose than the parental compound; this effect could be understandable because IFC-305 presented a delay in the maximal absorption than adenosine (20 vs. 30 min), but adenosine level rapidly declined to practically undetectable levels between 60 and 120 min, while IFC-305 presented a significant liver concentration even 120 min after its administration; this behavior could be explained by a 20% diminution of the activity of the adenosine deaminase, in the presence of IFC-305, an enzyme responsible to transform adenosine to inosine. These results suggest that IFC-305 clearance is much slower than that of adenosine [33]. With these results, we decided to explore the hepatoprotective properties of this adenosine compound, treating rats (50 mg/kg body weight, three times per week) during 5 weeks after cirrhosis induction with CCl_4.

Cirrhotic rats treated with IFC-305 present a healthy-like liver phenotype compared with cirrhotic rats and also with cirrhotic rats treated with saline during 5 weeks after cirrhosis induction. Besides, decreased fibrosis was evident in response to IFC-305 treatment, accelerating fibrosis resolution, leaving only 4% of fibrotic area, while increasing parenchymal liver area from 87 to 90%, and collagen was decreased to half-level as compared to saline-treated rats. This improvement in liver architecture was in accordance with liver physiological amelioration; IFC-305 reduced significantly bilirubin and serum transaminase activities [17], and ATP levels were equivalent to those of healthy liver [34], corroborating that IFC-305 presents the same hepatoprotective properties reverting cirrhosis than adenosine but with a lower dose.

3. Cell cycle inhibition during cirrhosis and its recovery by IFC-305

Liver has a well-known capability to regenerate after resection [35]; the severity of liver fibrosis is considered to be related with impaired regenerative capacity, suggesting the arrest of cell cycle [36]. The fibrogenesis process is accompanied by energetic imbalance as well as oxidative damage generated by oxygen species that could result in chromosomal instability, which induces injury in the check points of the cellular cycle triggering an impaired regenerative capacity [34].

Cell cycle molecules play essential roles in hepatocyte proliferation. Specifically, G1-phase related molecules are important because they are a requisite to enter into cell cycle from quiescent state [34]. Considering adenosine is able to increase DNA synthesis as well as the mitotic index and the expression of proliferating cell nuclear antigen (PCNA) in a pre-established cirrhosis [31], over and above accelerating progression of cell cycle during liver regeneration in rats subjected to one-third hepatectomy [37], we have explored cell cycle state during cirrhosis and changes mediated by IFC-305.

During cirrhosis, there is no evident change on PCNA, which is an auxiliary protein of DNA polymerase delta and is an excellent marker of cell proliferation and it is present at the beginning of the S phase; but IFC-305 treatment generates a 10-fold increase of this protein, supporting the effect on proliferation activation mediated by this compound; this result was validated by immunohistochemistry [34]. Regarding cell cycle cyclins, cyclin D1 levels in cirrhotic state was not altered, but treatment with IFC-305 showed a 77% protein increase; this behavior correlates with expression levels of that cyclin. On the other hand, Cyclin B1 did not change in cirrhotic rats, but IFC-305 treatment reduces by 30% the protein level [34]. Cyclin D1 belongs to G1 phase and is fundamental to initiate cell cycle and requires the association with cyclin-dependent kinase 4 or 6 (CDK4/CDK6) to form an active complex and allows the progression of cell cycle to S phase, whereas degradation of cyclin B1 is important for metaphase-anaphase transition and progression of cell cycle [38]. Evaluating the levels of CDK4, we did not find changes in cirrhosis but IFC-305 generates a high increment of this protein. In the case of CDK6, the protein is present in cirrhosis, the cessation of CCl_4 and saline solution administration reduces its levels, meanwhile IFC-305 treatment maintains elevated the presence of CDK6 [33]. These results suggest that both CDK4 and CDK6 could form a complex with Cyclin D1 and favor cell cycle progress in response to IFC-305 treatment. The complex Cyclin D/CDK4/6 is responsible for Rb protein phosphorylation, promoting the release of E2F1, which can induce transcription of several genes involved in cell cycle entry into S phase and induction or inhibition of apoptosis [39]. In livers from cirrhotic rats, there is a reduction of phospho-Rb (Ser 795), and IFC-305 restores the healthy levels; *Rb* gene expression correlates with protein levels. Analysis of E2F1 protein levels reveals a decrease of this protein in cirrhotic livers and administration with saline solution during 5 weeks after cirrhosis inductions partially reestablishes the levels of that protein but IFC-305 generates a higher increment than the one reached with saline; this increment together with Rb gain supports the reactivation of cell cycle, suggesting the entry to S phase of cell cycle [34].

Another level to regulate cell cycle progression is related with its inhibitors; with regard to this, p21 is reduced 40% in cirrhotic animals and IFC-305 is able to reassemble the healthy liver levels; p27, another cell cycle inhibitor, did not show effects that could be related with cirrhosis establishment neither to IFC-305 treatment during 5 weeks [34], so it is possible to suggest that one of the key cell cycle inhibitors in cirrhosis development is p21.

Trying to understand which could be the signal that generates this reactivation of cell cycle, we evaluated hepatocyte growth factor (HGF) levels in serum and liver; HGF originally identified and cloned as a potent mitogen for hepatocytes, is a strong protective and trophic factor for many tissues and organs [40]. Since HGF is produced mainly by mesenchymal cells and c-Met, its specific receptor tyrosine kinase is expressed in most epithelial, endothelial, and somatic stem cells [41]. In cirrhosis, there is a little increment of HGF in serum but in liver, there are no significant changes; meanwhile, rats treated with IFC-305 trigger a threefold increase of serum HGF versus healthy animals and a 35% increase versus cirrhotic animals; in liver, there is a trend to increase the levels of HGF compared with both healthy and cirrhotic rats. On the other hand, c-Met receptors present a 25% increase in cirrhotic animals with further increase after 5 weeks of progress, but treatment with IFC-305 induced a diminution in relation with cirrhotic rats administered with saline [34]. With these results, we could suggest that IFC-305 is able to increase HGF levels in serum of cirrhotic rats, which could interact with c-Met in liver, being the mitogenic signal which could trigger the reactivation of cell cycle recovery.

4. Inflammation, the beginning of liver disease and a key of IFC-305-mediated cirrhosis resolution

In recent years, it has been demonstrated that the immune response is one of the main mechanisms involved in the progression and repair of liver pathologies [42].

Liver injuries provide a proper model of inflammation and repair, showing a complex interaction of parenchymal, no-parenchymal cells and the extracellular matrix, all of them, components of the mammalian wound-healing response. In almost all etiologies, cirrhosis is preceded by fibrosis and inflammation, with elements of innate and adaptive immune response that are crucial in regulating these processes [43]. Recent efforts to confront these fibrotic diseases are focused on finding specific marks that transform an acute inflammation to a chronic one, and to use them as therapeutic aims for treatment and reversion of this phenomenon [44]. The immune response plays an essential role in this transformation, mainly by diverse cellular phenotypes [45]. The participation of immune cells, such as Kupffer cells (KCs), the liver macrophages, as initial effectors, is one of the main responsible of cirrhosis development [46, 47]. They are antigen presenting cells and represent an immune cell population related to liver fibrosis treatment.

The KCs present diverse activation phenotypes: M1 related to inflammation and M2 anti-inflammation related with resolution of inflammation processes [48–50], both are regulated by extracellular signals such as adenosine [51] and are directly connected with other immune cells types as B and T cells.

In liver diseases, the phenomenon, in a canonical way, occurs when the activated KCs regulate the hepatic stellate cells and other molecular and cell interactions associated with the establishment of cirrhosis [52, 53]. KCs also interact with other cells, like neutrophils, hepatocytes, etc., mainly through molecules directly associated with inflammation, tissue damage, and fibrosis, like cytokines and chemokines, such as IL-1β, IL-6, TNF-α, and MCP-1 [54] or ROS (reactive oxygen species) which promote the inflammatory response; KCs could be contributing to anti-inflammatory effects with IL-10 and other cytokines involved in tissue repair [55]. The liver is the main organ that produces and removes cytokines; all cell types in the liver are capable of cytokine production, parenchymal and non-parenchymal cells [56, 57].

By their destructiveness, macrophages guide the course of the inflammatory response and are involved in the synthesis and repair of damaged tissue during the inflammatory process, participating actively in the resolution of inflammation [58]. There are two proposed macrophage subtypes; activated by two ways: the classical pathway (M1) or the alternative pathway (M2) [59]. These different polarization states will depend on the microenvironment and the source of damage that has occurred. The classical activation is critical for the initiation and maintenance of the inflammatory process and to the response against pathogens and immune response.

Classical activation or M1 is produced by the interaction of TLR4 receptor with PAMPs such as LPS, from Gram-negative bacteria wall or by specific cytokines such as TNF-α or γ-IFN. This group of classically activated macrophages produces large amounts of proinflammatory cytokines such as TNF-α, interleukins (IL-1β, IL-6, and IL-12), proinflammatory chemokines such as MCP-1, and nitric oxide (NO), promoting activation, migration of other cells, and tissue damage [58].

In the case of alternative activation, the Th2 cells secrete cytokines such as IL-4 or IL-13 and induce the macrophage alternative M2 phenotype [60]. These M2 macrophages have very little capacity to present antigens while secrete high levels of anti-inflammatory cytokines such as IL-10. Unlike classical activation, these macrophages are not able to produce nitric oxide from L-arginine and also fail to control the growth of intracellular pathogens [61]. However, they are capable of producing a high quantity of arginase 1 enzyme that metabolizes L-arginine to produce proline, glutamate, and polyamines promoting tissue repair [62].

We have demonstrated that in the experimental model of CCl_4-induced cirrhosis, the IFC-305 treatment generates several changes in the inflammatory process, mediated by cytokines and immune cells [63]. During the development of cirrhosis, we observed an increment in the liver inflammatory cytokines, IL-6, IL-1β, MCP-1, and TNF-α, in plasma and liver tissue, as well as an increment of M1 macrophages (CD163+/CD11b+). The IFC-305 treatment decreased these inflammatory cytokines, reduced the M1 inflammatory macrophages, and increased the M2 anti-inflammatory macrophages (HIS36+/CD11b+). The anti-inflammatory role of IFC-305 was also supported by elevation of IL-10, an enhanced metabolic activity of arginase, reduction of NO levels in serum rats, a diminution of the protein levels of inducible nitric oxide synthetase, and an increment of the protein levels of arginase 1 in the liver. These results suggest that the IFC-305 modulates the immune response in cirrhosis and supports the hepatic protective action through an anti-inflammatory role, mainly mediated by Kupffer cells [64].

5. Hepatic stellate cells, generators of extracellular matrix components which trigger fibrosis and its activation prevention by IFC-305

Liver fibrosis is characterized by an accumulation of collagen types I and III that are secreted by liver myofibroblast. These cells are originated mainly from hepatic stellate cells (HSCs) and in a less number from the periportal fibroblast or bone marrow cells. In normal liver, HSCs represent almost 10% of all resident cells of the liver. They are quiescent cells specialized in lipid storage, mostly retinyl esters. When there is a liver damage, the HSC become activated or transdifferentiate to myofibroblast phenotype, characterized for being proliferative, pro-inflammatory, and contractile and for increased synthesis of ECM proteins [65].

The activation of HSCs is promoted by stimuli from resident and infiltrating inflammatory cells that produce fibrogenic, proliferative, and inflammatory cytokines such as TGF-β, PDGF, and TNF-α, among others, in addition to reactive oxygen species [65].

In order to clarify the hepatoprotector role of IFC-305 in the CCl_4-induced liver fibrosis at a molecular and cellular level, we explored the effect of IFC-305 on the activation of HSCs. These cells isolated from normal rat livers become activated *in vitro* after 7 days in culture, in a similar manner that occurs *in vivo* after a liver injury. We isolated HSCs from normal rat livers and cultured them for 7 days. We found that IFC-305 treatment suppresses their activation, determined by the inhibition of *Col1a1* mRNA expression, prevention of Rho activation, inhibition of

PDGF-stimulated proliferation, and increased expression of anti-fibrogenic genes such as *Pparg*, *Smad7*, and *Mmp-13* [66].

Hepatic fibrosis is characterized by ECM deposition, specially the type I collagen protein. The excess of ECM is due to an imbalance between its production and its degradation. ECM degradation is carried out by matrix metalloproteinases (MMPs), whose activity is negatively regulated by tissue inhibitors of matrix metalloproteinases (TIMPs). During progression of liver fibrosis, activated HSCs produce an excess of ECM and increase the expression of TIMP-1 and TIMP-2, resulting in an excess of ECM deposition. In rodents, the MMP-13 is the principal matrix metalloproteinase that degrades type I collagen [67]. Treatment of HSCs with IFC-305 inhibited the production of *Col1a1* mRNA but also increased the expression of *Mmp13* mRNA, which may result in an important decrease of collagen deposition.

The main fibrogenic cytokine is TGF-β, which signals into the cell through membrane kinase TGF-type I and type II receptors, which activate the intracellular Smad proteins and transduce the TGF-α signal to the nucleus. The Smad 7 acts as a negative regulator of this pathway [65]. The *Smad7* mRNA expression induced by IFC-305 could result in the inhibition of TGF-β signaling and inhibition of HSC activation.

Peroxisome Proliferator Activated Receptor gamma (PPARγ) regulates cellular fatty acid storage and adipogenesis of fibroblast. Another very important effect of IFC-305 on HSC is an increase of *Pparg* mRNA expression. PPARγ is expressed in quiescent HSC, and its expression is rapidly decreased during HSC activation *in vitro* and *in vivo* [68]. It is well documented that expression of PPARγ or treatment with its natural or synthetic ligands inhibits HSC activation or can reverse the activated HSC phenotype to the quiescent one [69]. The increased expression of *Pparg* mRNA with IFC305 in HSCs could be contributing to maintain their quiescent phenotype.

The IFC-305 also inhibited the PDGF-BB-stimulated proliferation of HSC; exploring the mechanism, we found that this effect was independent of adenosine receptors, but required their uptake into cells by adenosine transporters followed by their intracellular conversion to AMP by adenosine kinase, leading to increased levels of AMP, pyrimidine starvation, and inhibition of DNA synthesis [66].

In summary, we demonstrated that HSCs are an important target of the anti-fibrotic role of IFC-305 contributing to its hepatoprotective effect on liver fibrosis.

6. Gene expression deregulation in cirrhosis and IFC-305 modulation beyond genetics

With the interest to have a general view of molecular changes occurring in cirrhosis, we assessed the transcriptome evaluation of both cirrhotic and cirrhotic livers treated with IFC-305 and found 413 deregulated genes in cirrhosis, and IFC-305 treatment reduces the genes with deregulated expression to 263; making a gene ontology, we noticed that the highest proportion of deregulated genes is related with signal transduction, and interestingly, some of these deregulated genes are involved in TGF-β signaling pathway, lipid metabolism, urea cycle, and fibrogenesis.

Validating some of these differential expressed genes, we found an over-expression of *Fn1* (fibronectin 1) and *Col1a1* in cirrhosis; both of them are regulated by TGF-β signaling pathway, and importantly, *Col1a1* gene encodes a component of type I collagen called the pro-α1(I) chain that constitutes one of the main ECM proteins in the fibrotic liver. In fact, expression of *Tgfb1* gene was also increased in cirrhosis, and other two genes with the same behavior were the complement *C9* and

Apoa1 [17]. PPARγ has anti-fibrogenic activity inhibiting collagen I transcription [70]; there was a reduction in transcript levels of *Pparg* gene in cirrhosis state, in concordance with other reports [71, 72]. Transcriptome analysis also revealed three genes involved in ornithine and urea metabolism; the transcript level of *Ass1* gene was reduced as well as *Cps1* gene. Making a deeper analysis of the transcriptome data, we could identify a chromatin-related gene deregulated in cirrhosis; *HDAC3* histone deacetylase is over-expressed during cirrhosis. IFC-305 is able to reduce the levels to healthy-like levels for three fibrogenic genes (*Fn1*, *Col1a1*, and *Tgfb1*), *C9, Apob1* and *Hdac3;* meanwhile, this compound generates the increasing expression of *Pparg* and *Cps1* recovering the levels of the healthy liver and partially restoring the levels of *Ass1* [17]. Analyzing proteins, we could identify an increment in collagen I and HDAC3 and a reduction of PPARγ during cirrhosis, and the treatment with IFC-305 resembles the healthy-like levels of these three proteins [16]. Thus, through this quantitative analysis of expression and protein levels, IFC-305 shows capabilities to modulate the gene expression of some important genes involved in liver fibrogenesis.

During CCl_4-induced cirrhosis, besides hepatocellular damage previously mentioned, there is chromosome instability [73] that could be induced by hypomethylation on DNA, and contributes to carcinogenesis [74]. Considering cirrhosis as a pre-neoplastic state (because 80% of hepatocellular carcinoma cases are preceded by cirrhosis) [11], it is possible that the big changes in gene expression could be directed by chromosomal instability generated by CCl_4, but beyond the genetic alterations that probably are occurring, many of these changes could be related to regulation of gene expression at epigenetic level even more because chromosomal instability could be occurring by DNA hypomethylation. Also, it is important to remember that HDAC3 was incremented in cirrhosis, so some changes in gene expression could also be modified by changes in chromatin.

Every process which is able to influence in heritable gene expression without affecting DNA sequence is considered as an epigenetic regulation process [75]. DNA methylation is probably the most studied epigenetic modification [76, 77]; it consists in the incorporation of methyl group in 5 position of cytosine from CpG dinucleotide. This incorporation does not modify DNA sequence and can influence directly in transcriptional activity [78]. Methylated DNA distribution along genome shows an enrichment on noncoding regions, repetitive elements [75], and further, it inactivates mobile elements of the genome as transposons and sequences of viral origin, having a function in genome stability maintenance, blocking undesired recombination events [76]. On the other hand, on CpG islands of active genes, there is no enrichment of this DNA modification [75] and participates in permanent gene silencing in different steps of development [78, 79]. DNA methylation is directed by DNA methyltransferase enzymes which use S-adenosylmethionine (SAM) as methyl donor from methionine cycle and the product of this reaction is S-adenosylhomocysteine (SAH). It is important to mention that one important factor to modulate biological methylation reactions (to DNA, RNA, proteins, and phospholipids) is the hepatocellular ratio SAM/SAH [80].

The discovery of an active DNA demethylation pathway that involves the conversion of 5mC to oxidized forms, like 5hmC, by DNA dioxygenases TETs and DNA repair through the base excision system, incorporates a dynamic reversibility of DNA methylation [81–84]. Ever since the discovery of this dynamics, strenuous efforts have been made to characterize the precise role of 5hmC; such roles are becoming more evident as we learn about 5hmC-specific genomic localization, its relative stability, and recognition by other proteins [85], and current studies have shown that this DNA modification has an antagonic role to 5mC [86].

We have previously shown that adenosine can modulate trans-methylation reactions, like methylation of phospholipids, via regulation of

S-adenosylmethionine (SAM) levels [87], so that we make an approach to SAM levels and found that during cirrhosis, the amount of this molecule is diminished, whereas IFC-305 treatment restored the physiological levels; this suggests that during cirrhosis, it could be an imbalance of methylation reactions, and IFC-305, like adenosine, could also regulate this process [16].

Epigenetic changes in cirrhosis are little understood; some studies demonstrated a reduction on DNA methylation through the genome in CCl_4-induced cirrhosis [15, 88], and analyzing in a global way this modification, we obtained the same behavior. With these results and in order to assess DNA methylation dynamics, 5hmC levels were measured and a similar behavior to the one observed with 5mC, a reduction of 5hmC in cirrhosis in concordance with group of Mann findings, was found [89]. Treatment with IFC-305 triggers a regaining of both 5mC and 5hmC [16]. These results together suggest that there is a perturbation of DNA methylation dynamic during cirrhosis, while IFC-305 is able to modulate this dynamic, possibly reducing chromosome instability.

Another level of epigenetic regulation is related with genome packaging in chromatin, which has a direct repercussion in transcriptional activity, being mandatory its remodeling, space specifically, and in a time defined way to carry out gene expression [90]. Histones are a fundamental component of chromatin structure, being a target of a big variety of post-translational modifications (PTMs), which allows the formation of particular and regulated chromatin states; furthermore these modifications could be inherited post-mitotically [91]. We want to highlight among histone PTMs, lysine acetylation. DNA association with histone *core* is facilitated by electrical charge difference between both molecules, but histone acetylation neutralizes lysine positive charge, weakening nucleosome-DNA interaction and triggering a less compact conformation which favors transcription [92].

Considering the finding that histone deacetylase HDAC3 level was high during cirrhosis, global histone H4 acetylation was assessed, finding a reduction in this histone PTM in cirrhotic livers. Physiological levels of global histone H4 acetylation in cirrhotic rats treated with IFC-305 were recovered [16]. Together, these results suggest that deregulated gene expression during cirrhosis could be related with epigenetic deregulation involving DNA methylation dynamics and changes in histone acetylation; besides, IFC-305 has epigenetic properties being able to modulate 5mC, 5hmC, and histone H4 acetylation in a global way, favoring the recovery of physiological levels of each epigenetic modification and triggering the rescue of healthy-like gene expression in liver.

7. Getting deeper into cirrhosis resolution or epigenetic regulation of *Pparg* and *Col1a1* by IFC-305

Once established that IFC-305 is able to reverse fibrosis, reactivating cell cycle progression in cirrhotic livers, favoring an anti-inflammatory environment, blocking hepatic stellate cell activation, and regulating gene expression through epigenetic modulation, we analyzed the regulation of two of the main genes with modified expression during cirrhosis, *Pparg* and *Col1a1*. Reminding, collagen I is the mayor ECM protein and responsible for liver fibrosis, *Col1a1*, a gene which encodes pro-α1 chain of this protein is over-regulated in cirrhosis, and there is a reduction of nuclear receptor PPARγ in this pathological condition.

PPARγ has antifibrotic properties because it is able to inhibit collagen I gene transcription. This inhibition is mediated by the ability of nuclear receptor to compete with NF-I/p300 association to the *Col1a1* gene in HSC [70]. p300 has a histone acetyltransferase activity that transfers an acetyl group to the lysine residue

[93] generating an open chromatin context in *Col1a1* gene promoter favoring its expression; whether PPARγ replaces p300 in Col1a1 gene promoter, there is a chromatin context change because of the loss of acetylation activity in this region, and the consequent blocking of the gene expression.

On the other hand, regulation of *Pparg* expression is directed by MeCP2 protein in HSC activation like in cirrhosis. MeCP2 binds to regulatory regions of the gene which are CpG enriched and recruits histone H3K9me3 writer enzymes suppressing initial transcription of the gene. Furthermore, MeCP2 is required for polycomb repressor complex 2 EZH2 component that establishes histone H3K27me mark on the downstream coding gene region, blocking transcription elongation [94]. This mechanism could explain the reduction of PPARγ levels in cirrhosis and therefore the over-expression of *Col1a1* in cirrhosis.

Considering that MeCP2 is a methyl binding protein [94], DNA methylation state was evaluated with sodium bisulfite DNA modification on *Pparg* gene promoter, and it was found that both healthy and cirrhotic livers present *Pparg* gene promoter without DNA methylation, and IFC-305 treatment does not modify this nonmethylated state [16]. Evaluating histone H4 acetylation and histone H3K27me3 on *Pparg* gene promoter through chromatin immunoprecipitation assay, we found that in cirrhosis, there is a trend to compact chromatin context mainly dictated by histone H4 acetylation reduction, which correlates with decreased expression and protein levels; after treatment with IFC-305 chromatin, there is an open chromatin context on *Pparg* gene promoter triggered by an increase on histone H4 acetylation and a reduction of histone H3K27me3, going hand by hand with over-expression and increase of protein levels [16]. These findings suggest that reduction of PPARγ on cirrhosis is coordinated by a chromatin compaction on gene promoter, and IFC-305 treatment generates a decompaction of gene promoter with the consequent increase of gene expression.

The next step was to identify if IFC-305 mediated fibrosis reversion is related with *Col1a1* gene expression blocking though PPARγ was to assess nuclear receptor deposition on *Col1a1* gene promoter, but we were not able to find an increment of this interaction in whole cirrhotic tissues treated with IFC-305; rather, we found a diminishment of PPARγ deposition [16]. Further experiments on isolated HSCs treated with IFC-305 are required to know if this molecular mechanism is occurring directly in responsible cells of fibrosis generation. So, we asses DNA methylation state on *Col1a1* gene promoter, to know if this epigenetic mechanism is involved in regulation of gene expression during cirrhosis. In healthy liver, *Col1a1* gene promoter presents a methylated state, which correlates with the absence of collagen I overproduction; in cirrhosis state and progress of the illness, there is an important reduction on methylation state on *Col1a1* gene promoter going hand by hand with accumulation of collagen I; and finally, treatment with IFC-305 generates a remethylation of gene promoter and an enrichment of methylation around transcription start site, associated with collagen reduction.

With these results, we could propose that fibrosis generation could be directed by loss of DNA methylation on *Col1a1* gene promoter, and one of the mechanisms of action that could explain cirrhosis resolution mediated by IFC-305 is the modulation of DNA methylation on *Col1a1* gene.

Blocking the prelude of hepatocellular carcinoma, a key point to avoid chronic liver injury progress.

Along this chapter, some cellular and molecular alterations that characterize cirrhosis have been described: a pathology that results in the combination of factors which alters liver environment, beginning with an immunological response originated by macrophages inflammatory polarization that triggers hepatic stellate cell activation, with alterations at chromatin level resulting in chromosome instability and altered gene expression favoring the fibrogenic process. All these changes, as a whole, could facilitate progress of the illness to hepatocellular carcinoma (HCC), which is the most common primary carcinoma of the liver. Up to 85% of HCC cases arise in chronically inflamed and subsequently cirrhotic livers [95].

According to GLOBOCAN-IARC datasets [96], liver cancer is estimated to be at the 7th place of cancer incidence and the 4th cancer death cause in 2018. Considering cirrhosis as a prelude of HCC, it is understandable that many liver cancers follow a pattern of pathologic evolution, starting from cirrhosis to low-grade dysplastic nodules, high-grade dysplastic nodules, early HCC, progressed HCC and, finally to advance HCC. Furthermore, this progress of illness involves a more evident imbalance between genetic and epigenetic factors; regarding genetic ones, early dysplastic nodules present a genome with a very limited genetic variation, while advanced HCC has a heterogeneous genome with a range of 72–182 mutations [97, 98]. On the other hand, concerning epigenetic aspects, a genome-wide DNA hypomethylation in HCC has been described, which could be indicative of poor survival [99]. In the same sense, another study described that aberrantly methylated differential expressed genes are related with cell cycle progress, p53 signaling, and MAPK signaling in HCC [100]. Alteration on DNA methylation state could be explained by down-regulation of TET dioxygenases in HCC condition with the consequent reduction of 5hmC levels [101]. In normal tissue there is a characteristic difference between euchromatic and heterochromatic regions that is lost in cancer condition; it has been suggested that lost could be generated by a reduction of 5hmC levels which goes around 70%. Furthermore, the specific relationship between 5hmC and chromatin marks in normal tissue is largely erased in tumors and suggests that 5hmC landscape change in cancer could be associated with chromatin structure alterations and deregulation of gene expression during tumorigenesis [102].

HCC may progress silently in patients with sufficient liver function; due to vague complaints and nonspecific symptoms, HCC diagnosis is usually delayed [103]. Selected patients with localized disease may be treated with curative intents with resection, liver transplantation, or local therapy like radial frequency ablation, chemoembolization or radio-embolization. However, the majority of patients with HCC are not candidates for resection [104, 105]. For patients suffering from advanced HCC, chemotherapy failed to demonstrate a survival advantage [106, 107]; so far, sorafenib is the first and only target orientated agent approved as therapy of HCC [105], but it only extends survival of patients with advanced stage disease for 3 months, and this medication causes considerable adverse events and offers no symptom palliation [108]. This lack of effective treatment and surgical impediment highlights the importance to reinforce molecular target therapies.

Preclinical studies indicated that IFC-305 is not toxic, neither genotoxic, nor teratogenic and it is anti-carcinogenic [33]. Considering this last property, we assessed IFC-305 effects on a chronic model of liver intoxication with diethylnitrosamine and found that it could act as a HCC chemopreventive agent [109, 110]. The above suggests that some anti-fibrotic effects of the compound could prevent cancer development, being an adjuvant in chronic liver disease treatment. Currently we are studying a deep molecular level to identify IFC-305 mechanism of action in prevention of cancer establishment and potential disease reversion.

Considering recent advances in cirrhosis knowledge, we could suggest that in the not long future, drugs targeting specific molecular keys for cirrhotic and HCC will be developed and potentially they could be the first line of treatment even after surgery.

8. Conclusion

Cirrhosis is a complex pathology, which involves deregulation at different levels (**Figure 1**); some insults such as hepatitis viral infections, alcohol, high fat diet, or even self-immune events could trigger the development of the illness, denoted by biochemical alterations like albumin reduction and increase of transaminases. In our case, we assessed the study of this disease using CCl_4, which generates hepatocellular damage. Once cell membrane is affected by free radicals from CCl_4 metabolism, through epoxide formation, KCs are activated to phagocytose damaged cells; this activation causes an inflammatory process, due to M1 macrophage activation. Whether this inflammation is perpetuated, HSCs could be activated, becoming the main producers of fibrosis (**Figure 1B**). At molecular level, cirrhotic-damaged liver loses the capability to proliferate; there is a reduction in DNA methylation, 5hmC, and histone H4 acetylation, which generates chromosome instability and therefore alteration of gene expression, affecting principally fibrogenic genes. Among important genes involved in the fibrogenic process are *Pparg* and *Col1a1*. Cirrhotic liver presents a compact chromatin context of *Pparg* gene promoter with the consequent reduction of both its transcript and protein; on the other hand, *Col1a1* gene promoter loses DNA methylation, and this correlates with gene overexpression and the increment of protein levels. Adenosine derivative, IFC-305, has hepatoprotective properties (**Figure 1C**); it is able to reduce fibrosis, ameliorate parenchymal area and recover liver function. Treatment with this compound polarizes the macrophages to an anti-inflammatory phenotype M2, increasing the levels of immunosuppressant cytokine IL-10 and arginase 1; the reduction of the inflammatory process facilitates the inhibition of HSC activation and the consequent reduction of fibrosis. At molecular level, high serum levels of HGF, principal liver mitogen, could interact with elevated levels of its receptor, c-Met, and stimulate cell cycle progression, providing once more the regenerative capacity to the liver. IFC-305 could favor a genome instability diminishment as a consequence of the

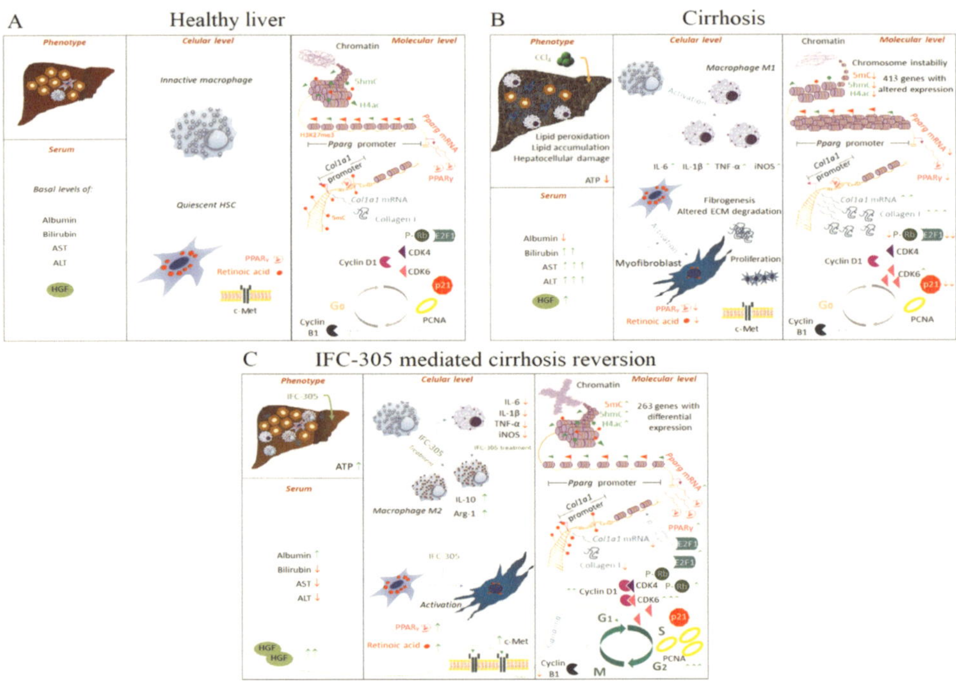

Figure 1.
Architectural, physiological, cellular, and molecular alteration during CCl_4-induced cirrhosis and hepatoprotective effects of IFC-305. We show four different analyzed levels in this section: phenotype, denoting architecture and cell composition of the liver; Serum, biochemical markers related with liver function; cellular level, changes found in non-parenchymal cells; molecular level, changes in cell cycle components, chromatin, and gene expression. (A) Healthy liver; (B) CCl_4-induced cirrhosis state; (C) pre-established cirrhosis treated with IFC-305.

reestablishment of DNA methylation levels and 5hmC and Histone H4 acetylation; these effects on chromatin trigger the recovery of healthy-like gene expression. Fibrosis resolution mediated by IFC-305 could be explained by the generation of an open chromatin context of *Pparg* gene promoter that correlates with its gene and protein up-regulation. High levels of PPARγ could act as a repressor of *Col1a1* expression in HSC; on the other hand, *Col1a1* gene promoter gains DNA methylation on promoter and TSS, this methylation state goes hand by hand with reduction of collagen I expression and protein, favoring a decrease in fibrosis, a key point in cirrhosis resolution. These studies support molecules and cell behavior modified by IFC-305 as a potential target for new drugs to treat cirrhosis, contribute to the understanding of liver fibrosis at epigenetic level, open the door to the exploration of chromatin modifications as a potential biomarker for early detection and intervention of liver diseases, and support the use of IFC-305 as therapy for liver illness. Finally, we highlight the relationship between cirrhosis and HCC, how liver fibrosis is the prelude of HCC and in what manner IFC-305 could be an adjuvant preventing HCC by its anti-cirrhotic and anti-neoplastic effects, and how recent advances could favor development of an effective treatment, preferring a less invasive to surgical one.

Acknowledgements

This work has been supported by DGAPA-UNAM, grant numbers: IN214419 to VCS and IN203917 to FRT; CONACyT, México, grant: *Fronteras de la Ciencia* 290 to FRT; *Fundación Miguel Alemán, México "Estímulo a Investigaciones Médicas"* to VCS; PhD Fellowships from CONACyT: CVU 508509 to JRRA, CVU 298432 to RPCV, CVU 580148 to NGC. We acknowledge the assistance of Rosario Pérez-Molina, Georgina Guerrero-Avendaño, Fernando Suaste-Olmos, Enrique Chávez, Rosario Villaseñor Ávila, and Gabriela Valdés Silva.

Conflict of interest

The authors declare no conflict of interest.

Nomenclature

5hmC	5-hydroximethylcytosine
5-LO	5-lipoxygenase
5mC	5-methylcytosine
ALT	alanine aminotransferase
AMP	adenosine monophosphate
AST	aspartate aminotransferase
ATP	adenosine triphosphate
$CCl_3\cdot$	trichloromethane radical
$CCl_3OO\cdot$	trichloromethyl peroxy radical
CCl_4	carbon tetrachloride
CDK4	cyclin-dependent kinase (for example, CDK4, CDK6, etc.)
c-Met	tyrosine-protein kinase Met or hepatocyte growth factor receptor
Col1a1	type I collagen pro-α1(I) chain gene
CpG	cytosine guanine dinucleotide
DNA	deoxyribonucleic acid

E2F1	transcription factor E2F1
ECM	extracellular matrix
H3K27me3	histone H3 trimethyl lysine 27
H4ac	hyperacetylated histone H4
HCC	hepatocellular carcinoma
HDAC	histone deacetylase
HGF	hepatocyte growth factor
HSC	hepatic stellate cells
IFC-305	aspartate salt of adenosine: 2-aminosuccinic acid–2-(6-amino-9H-purin-9-yl)-5-(hydroxymethyl)tetrahydrofuran-3,4-diol (1:1)
IL	interleukin (for example, IL-1β, IL-10, etc.)
iNOS	inducible nitric oxide synthase
KC	Kupffer cells
LPS	lipopolysaccharide
M1	inflammatory macrophages
M2	anti-inflammatory macrophages
MAPK	mitogen-activated protein kinase
MCP-1α	macrophage protein inflammatory 1-alpha
MeCP2	methyl-CpG binding protein 2
MMP9	matrix metalloproteinase 9
mRNA	messenger ribonucleic acid
NO	nitric oxide
p21	cyclin-dependent kinase inhibitor 1
p27	cyclin-dependent kinase inhibitor 1B
P450	CYP450 cytochrome
PAMPs	pathogen associated molecular patterns
PCNA	proliferating cell nuclear antigen
PDGF	platelet-derived growth factor
PPARγ	peroxisome proliferator-activated receptor gamma
PTMs	post-translational modifications
Rb	retinoblastoma protein
RNA	ribonucleic acid
ROS	reactive oxygen species
SAH	S-adenosylhomocysteine
SAM	S-adenosylmethionine
STAT6	signal transducer and activator of transcription 6
TET	DNA dioxygenase ten-eleven translocation
TGF-β	transforming growth factor beta
TIMPs	tissue inhibitors of matrix metalloproteinases
TLR4	Toll-like receptor 4
TNF-α	tumoral necrosis factor alpha
VEGF	vascular endothelial growth factor
α-SMA	alpha smooth muscle actin.

Author details

Jesús Rafael Rodríguez-Aguilera[1], Rebeca Pérez-Cabeza de Vaca[1,2], Nuria Guerrero-Celis[1], Gabriela Velasco-Loyden[1], Mariana Domínguez-López[1], Félix Recillas-Targa[3] and Victoria Chagoya de Sánchez[1]*

1 Department of Cell Biology and Development, Institute of Cellular Physiology, UNAM, Mexico City, Mexico

2 Coordination of Research, National Medical Center "20 de noviembre", ISSSTE, Mexico City, Mexico

3 Department of Molecular Genetics, Institute of Cellular Physiology, UNAM, Mexico City, Mexico

*Address all correspondence to: vchagoya@ifc.unam.mx

References

[1] Tsochatzis EA, Bosch J, Burroughs AK. Liver cirrhosis. Lancet. 2014;**383**: 1749-1761

[2] Ma C, Brunt EM. Histopathologic evaluation of liver biopsy for cirrhosis. Advances in Anatomic Pathology. 2012; **19**:220-230

[3] Fauci A, Kasper D, Longo D, Braunwald E, Hauser S, Jameson L, et al. Harrison Principios de Medicina Interna. 17th ed. China: McGraw-Hill/ Interamericana de México; 2009

[4] Chang TT, Liaw YF, Wu SS, Schiff E, Han KH, Lai CL, et al. Long-term entecavir therapy results in the reversal of fibrosis/cirrhosis and continued histological improvement in patients with chronic hepatitis B. Hepatology. 2010;**52**:886-893

[5] Chen G, Zhang L, Chen L, Wang H, Zhang Y, Bie P. Role of integrin alphavbeta6 in the pathogenesis of ischemia-related biliary fibrosis after liver transplantation. Transplantation. 2013;**95**:1092-1099

[6] Falize L, Guillygomarc'h A, Perrin M, Laine F, Guyader D, Brissot P, et al. Reversibility of hepatic fibrosis in treated genetic hemochromatosis: A study of 36 cases. Hepatology. 2006;**44**: 472-477

[7] Hammel P, Couvelard A, O'Toole D, Ratouis A, Sauvanet A, Flejou JF, et al. Regression of liver fibrosis after biliary drainage in patients with chronic pancreatitis and stenosis of the common bile duct. The New England Journal of Medicine. 2001;**344**:418-423

[8] Pol S, Carnot F, Nalpas B, Lagneau JL, Fontaine H, Serpaggi J, et al. Reversibility of hepatitis C virus-related cirrhosis. Human Pathology. 2004;**35**:107-112

[9] Wanless IR, Nakashima E, Sherman M. Regression of human cirrhosis. Morphologic features and the genesis of incomplete septal cirrhosis. Archives of Pathology and Laboratory Medicine. 2000;**124**:1599-1607

[10] Longo D, Kasper D, Jameson L, Fauci A, Hauser S, Loscalzo J. Harrison Principios de Medicina Interna. 18th ed. México: McGraw-Hill; 2012

[11] Forner A, Hessheimer AJ, Isabel Real M, Bruix J. Treatment of hepatocellular carcinoma. Critical Reviews in Oncology/Hematology. 2006;**60**:89-98

[12] Hernandez-Gea V, Friedman SL. Pathogenesis of liver fibrosis. Annual Review of Pathology. 2011;**6**:425-456

[13] Recillas-Targa F. Interdependency between genetic and epigenetic regulatory defects in cancer. Methods in Molecular Biology. 2014;**1165**:33-52

[14] Medina J. Medicina Ocupacional. Gases y Disolventes. 2011. Available from: http://es.scribd.com/doc/57239677/37/Tetracloruro-de-Carbono

[15] Varela-Moreiras G, Alonso-Aperte E, Rubio M, Gasso M, Deulofeu R, Alvarez L, et al. Carbon tetrachloride-induced hepatic injury is associated with global DNA hypomethylation and homocysteinemia: Effect of S-adenosylmethionine treatment. Hepatology. 1995;**22**:1310-1315

[16] Rodriguez-Aguilera JR, Guerrero-Hernandez C, Perez-Molina R, Cadena-Del-Castillo CE, Perez-Cabeza de Vaca R, Guerrero-Celis N, et al. Epigenetic effects of an adenosine derivative in a Wistar rat model of liver cirrhosis. Journal of Cellular Biochemistry. 2018; **119**:401-413

[17] Perez-Carreon JI, Martinez-Perez L, Loredo ML, Yanez-Maldonado L, Velasco-Loyden G, Vidrio-Gomez S,

et al. An adenosine derivative compound, IFC305, reverses fibrosis and alters gene expression in a pre-established CCl(4)-induced rat cirrhosis. The International Journal of Biochemistry and Cell Biology. 2010;**42**: 287-296

[18] Chagoya-de-Sánchez V, Suárez JA, Hernández-Muñoz R. Investigación y desarrollo de un fármaco para el tratamiento de la cirrosis. TIP Revista Especializada en Ciencias Químico-Biológicas. 2005;**8**:106-114

[19] Chagoya de Sanchez V, Brunner A, Pina E. In vivo modification of the energy charge in the liver cell. Biochemical and Biophysical Research Communications. 1972;**46**:1441-1445

[20] Chagoya de Sanchez V, Brunner A, Sanchez ME, Lopez C, Pina E. Utilization of adenosine as a tool in studies on the regulation of liver glycogen biosynthesis. Archives of Biochemistry and Biophysics. 1974;**160**: 145-150

[21] Garcia-Sainz JA, Hernandez-Munoz R, Santamaria A, de Sanchez VC. Mechanism of the fatty liver induced by cycloheximide and its reversibility by adenosine. Biochemical Pharmacology. 1979;**28**:1409-1413

[22] Hernandez-Munoz R, Santamaria A, Garcia-Sainz JA, Pina E, Chagoya de Sanchez V. On the mechanism of ethanol-induced fatty liver and its reversibility by adenosine. Archives of Biochemistry and Biophysics. 1978;**190**: 155-162

[23] Garcia-Sainz JA, Hernandez-Munoz R, Glender W, Pina E, Chagoya de Sanchez V. Effects of adenosine on ethanol-induced modifications of liver metabolism. Role of hepatic redox state, purine and fatty acid metabolism. Biochemical Pharmacology. 1980;**29**: 1709-1714

[24] Hernandez-Munoz R, Glender W, Diaz Munoz M, Adolfo J, Garcia-Sainz JA, Chagoya de Sanchez V. Effects of adenosine on liver cell damage induced by carbon tetrachloride. Biochemical Pharmacology. 1984;**33**:2599-2604

[25] Chagoya de Sanchez V, Hernandez-Munoz R, Yanez L, Vidrio S, Diaz-Munoz M. Possible mechanism of adenosine protection in carbon tetrachloride acute hepatotoxicity. Role of adenosine by-products and glutathione peroxidase. Journal of Biochemical Toxicology. 1995;**10**:41-50

[26] Hernandez-Munoz R, Diaz-Munoz M, Suarez J, Chagoya de Sanchez V. Adenosine partially prevents cirrhosis induced by carbon tetrachloride in rats. Hepatology. 1990;**12**:242-248

[27] Hernandez-Munoz R, Diaz-Munoz M, Chagoya de Sanchez V. Effects of adenosine administration on the function and membrane composition of liver mitochondria in carbon tetrachloride-induced cirrhosis. Archives of Biochemistry and Biophysics. 1992;**294**:160-167

[28] Hernandez-Munoz R, Diaz-Munoz M, Chagoya de Sanchez V. Possible role of cell redox state on collagen metabolism in carbon tetrachloride-induced cirrhosis as evidenced by adenosine administration to rats. Biochimica et Biophysica Acta. 1994; **1200**:93-99

[29] Hernandez-Munoz R, Chagoya de Sanchez V. In vivo correlation between liver and blood energy status as evidenced by chronic treatment of carbon tetrachloride and adenosine to rats. Canadian Journal of Physiology and Pharmacology. 1994;**72**:1252-1256

[30] Hernandez-Munoz R, Diaz-Munoz M, Lopez V, Lopez-Barrera F, Yanez L, Vidrio S, et al. Balance between oxidative damage and proliferative potential in an experimental rat model of CCl4-induced cirrhosis: Protective role of adenosine administration. Hepatology. 1997;**26**:1100-1110

[31] Hernandez-Munoz R, Diaz-Munoz M, Suarez-Cuenca JA, Trejo-Solis C, Lopez V, Sanchez-Sevilla L, et al. Adenosine reverses a preestablished CCl4-induced micronodular cirrhosis through enhancing collagenolytic activity and stimulating hepatocyte cell proliferation in rats. Hepatology. 2001; **34**:677-687

[32] Chagoya de Sanchez V. Circadian variations of adenosine and of its metabolism. Could adenosine be a molecular oscillator for circadian rhythms? Canadian Journal of Physiology and Pharmacology. 1995;**73**: 339-355

[33] Chagoya-de-Sánchez V, Hernández-Luis F, Díaz-Muñoz M, Hernández-Muñoz R. Role of the energy state of liver cell in cirrhosis development and treatment. In: Miranda LM, editor. Liver Cirrhosis Causes, Diagnosis and Treatment. New York, USA: Nova Science Publishers, Inc.; 2012. pp. 31-58

[34] Chagoya de Sanchez V, Martinez-Perez L, Hernandez-Munoz R, Velasco-Loyden G. Recovery of the cell cycle inhibition in CCl(4)-induced cirrhosis by the adenosine derivative IFC-305. International Journal of Hepatology. 2012;**2012**:212530

[35] Kokudo N, Kothary PC, Eckhauser FE, Raper SE. Transforming growth factor-alpha (TGF-alpha) improves hepatic DNA synthesis after hepatectomy in cirrhotic rats. Journal of Surgical Research. 1992;**52**:648-655

[36] Kato A, Bamba H, Shinohara M, Yamauchi A, Ota S, Kawamoto C, et al. Relationship between expression of cyclin D1 and impaired liver regeneration observed in fibrotic or cirrhotic rats. Journal of Gastroenterology and Hepatology. 2005; **20**:1198-1205

[37] Mendieta-Condado E, Pichardo-Olvera M, Sanchez-Sevilla L, Chagoya de Sanchez V, Hernandez-Munoz R. Adenosine administration accelerates progression of the cell cycle during rat liver regeneration induced by one-third hepatectomy. Journal of Pharmacology and Experimental Therapeutics. 2009; **331**:122-132

[38] Fung TK, Siu WY, Yam CH, Lau A, Poon RY. Cyclin F is degraded during G2-M by mechanisms fundamentally different from other cyclins. Journal of Biological Chemistry. 2002;**277**: 35140-35149

[39] Ertosun MG, Hapil FZ, Osman Nidai O. E2F1 transcription factor and its impact on growth factor and cytokine signaling. Cytokine and Growth Factor Reviews. 2016;**31**:17-25

[40] Bellan M, Castello LM, Pirisi M. Candidate biomarkers of liver fibrosis: A concise, pathophysiology-oriented Review. Journal of Clinical and Translational Hepatology. 2018;**6**: 317-325

[41] Fukushima T, Uchiyama S, Tanaka H, Kataoka H. Hepatocyte growth factor activator: A proteinase linking tissue injury with repair. International Journal of Molecular Sciences. 2018;**19**(11):3435

[42] Heymann F, Tacke F. Immunology in the liver—From homeostasis to disease. Nature Reviews. Gastroenterology and Hepatology. 2016; **13**:88-110

[43] Pellicoro A, Ramachandran P, Iredale JP, Fallowfield JA. Liver fibrosis and repair: Immune regulation of wound healing in a solid organ. Nature Reviews. Immunology. 2014;**14**:181-194

[44] Mallat A, Lotersztajn S. Cellular mechanisms of tissue fibrosis. 5. Novel insights into liver fibrosis. American Journal of Physiology. Cell Physiology. 2013;**305**:C789-C799

[45] Tacke F, Luedde T, Trautwein C. Inflammatory pathways in liver

homeostasis and liver injury. Clinical Reviews in Allergy and Immunology. 2009;**36**:4-12

[46] Muriel P, Escobar Y. Kupffer cells are responsible for liver cirrhosis induced by carbon tetrachloride. Journal of Applied Toxicology. 2003;**23**:103-108

[47] Edwards MJ, Keller BJ, Kauffman FC, Thurman RG. The involvement of Kupffer cells in carbon tetrachloride toxicity. Toxicology and Applied Pharmacology. 1993;**119**:275-279

[48] Dixon LJ, Barnes M, Tang H, Pritchard MT, Nagy LE. Kupffer cells in the liver. Comprehensive Physiology. 2013;**3**:785-797

[49] Ramachandran P, Iredale JP. Macrophages: Central regulators of hepatic fibrogenesis and fibrosis resolution. Journal of Hepatology. 2012; **56**:1417-1419

[50] Wan J, Benkdane M, Teixeira-Clerc F, Bonnafous S, Louvet A, Lafdil F, et al. M2 Kupffer cells promote M1 Kupffer cell apoptosis: A protective mechanism against alcoholic and nonalcoholic fatty liver disease. Hepatology. 2014;**59**: 130-142

[51] Hasko G, Cronstein B. Regulation of inflammation by adenosine. Frontiers in Immunology. 2013;**4**:85

[52] Kolios G, Valatas V, Kouroumalis E. Role of Kupffer cells in the pathogenesis of liver disease. World Journal of Gastroenterology. 2006;**12**:7413-7420

[53] Luckey SW, Petersen DR. Activation of Kupffer cells during the course of carbon tetrachloride-induced liver injury and fibrosis in rats. Experimental and Molecular Pathology. 2001;**71**:226-240

[54] Ramadori G, Armbrust T. Cytokines in the liver. European Journal of Gastroenterology and Hepatology. 2001; **13**:777-784

[55] Diehl AM. Cytokine regulation of liver injury and repair. Immunological Reviews. 2000;**174**:160-171

[56] Hsieh HG, Huang HC, Lee FY, Chan CY, Lee JY, Lee SD. Kinetics of cytokine expression in cirrhotic rats. Journal of the Chinese Medical Association. 2011; **74**:385-393

[57] Llorent L, Richaud-Patin Y, Alcocer-Castillejos N, Ruiz-Soto R, Mercado MA, Orozco H, et al. Cytokine gene expression in cirrhotic and non-cirrhotic human liver. Journal of Hepatology. 1996;**24**:555-563

[58] Laskin DL, Laskin JD. Role of macrophages and inflammatory mediators in chemically induced toxicity. Toxicology. 2001;**160**:111-118

[59] Traves PG, Luque A, Hortelano S. Macrophages, inflammation, and tumor suppressors: ARF, a new player in the game. Mediators of Inflammation. 2012; **2012**:568783

[60] Gordon S. Alternative activation of macrophages. Nature Reviews. Immunology. 2003;**3**:23-35

[61] Kropf P, Fuentes JM, Fahnrich E, Arpa L, Herath S, Weber V, et al. Arginase and polyamine synthesis are key factors in the regulation of experimental leishmaniasis in vivo. FASEB Journal. 2005;**19**:1000-1002

[62] Tsunawaki S, Sporn M, Ding A, Nathan C. Deactivation of macrophages by transforming growth factor-beta. Nature. 1988;**334**:260-262

[63] Pérez-Cabeza-de-Vaca R. “Efecto del hepatoprotector IFC-305 en las células de Kupffer en el modelo experimental de cirrosis inducida por CCl_4,” Maestría en Ciencias Bioquímicas, Biología Celular y Desarrollo. Instituto de Fisiología Celular: Universidad Nacional Autónoma de México, México; 2012

[64] Perez-Cabeza de Vaca R, Dominguez-Lopez M, Guerrero-Celis N, Rodriguez-Aguilera JR, Chagoya de Sanchez V. Inflammation is regulated by the adenosine derivative molecule, IFC-305, during reversion of cirrhosis in a CCl4 rat model. International Immunopharmacology. 2018;**54**:12-23

[65] Tsuchida T, Friedman SL. Mechanisms of hepatic stellate cell activation. Nature Reviews. Gastroenterology and Hepatology. 2017; **14**:397-411

[66] Velasco-Loyden G, Perez-Carreon JI, Aguero JF, Romero PC, Vidrio-Gomez S, Martinez-Perez L, et al. Prevention of in vitro hepatic stellate cells activation by the adenosine derivative compound IFC305. Biochemical Pharmacology. 2010;**80**: 1690-1699

[67] Schaefer B, Rivas-Estilla AM, Meraz-Cruz N, Reyes-Romero MA, Hernandez-Nazara ZH, Dominguez-Rosales JA, et al. Reciprocal modulation of matrix metalloproteinase-13 and type I collagen genes in rat hepatic stellate cells. The American Journal of Pathology. 2003;**162**:1771-1780

[68] Miyahara T, Schrum L, Rippe R, Xiong S, Yee HF Jr, Motomura K, et al. Peroxisome proliferator-activated receptors and hepatic stellate cell activation. The Journal of Biological Chemistry. 2000;**275**:35715-35722

[69] Hazra S, Xiong S, Wang J, Rippe RA, Krishna V, Chatterjee K, et al. Peroxisome proliferator-activated receptor gamma induces a phenotypic switch from activated to quiescent hepatic stellate cells. The Journal of Biological Chemistry. 2004;**279**: 11392-11401

[70] Yavrom S, Chen L, Xiong S, Wang J, Rippe RA, Tsukamoto H. Peroxisome proliferator-activated receptor gamma suppresses proximal alpha1(I) collagen promoter via inhibition of p300-facilitated NF-I binding to DNA in hepatic stellate cells. The Journal of Biological Chemistry. 2005;**280**: 40650-40659

[71] de Gottardi A, Pazienza V, Pugnale P, Bruttin F, Rubbia-Brandt L, Juge-Aubry CE, et al. Peroxisome proliferator-activated receptor-alpha and -gamma mRNA levels are reduced in chronic hepatitis C with steatosis and genotyp. 3 infection. Alimentary Pharmacology and Therapeutics. 2006; **23**:107-114

[72] Yang L, Chan CC, Kwon OS, Liu S, McGhee J, Stimpson SA, et al. Regulation of peroxisome proliferator-activated receptor-gamma in liver fibrosis. American Journal of Physiology. Gastrointestinal and Liver Physiology. 2006;**291**:G902-G911

[73] Michalopoulos GK. Liver regeneration: Molecular mechanisms of growth control. The FASEB Journal. 1990;**4**:176-187

[74] Hamilton JP. Epigenetics: Principles and practice. Digestive Diseases. 2011; **29**:130-135

[75] Allis CD, Jenuwein T, Reinberg D, Caparros ML. Epigenetics. New York, USA: Cold Spring Harbor Laboratory Press; 2007

[76] Bird A. DNA methylation patterns and epigenetic memory. Genes and Development. 2002;**16**:6-21

[77] Fullgrabe J, Kavanagh E, Joseph B. Histone onco-modifications. Oncogene. 2011;**30**:3391-3403

[78] Klose RJ, Bird AP. Genomic DNA methylation: The mark and its mediators. Trends in Biochemical Sciences. 2006;**31**:89-97

[79] Escamilla-Del-Arenal M, da Rocha ST, Heard E. Evolutionary diversity and developmental regulation of

X-chromosome inactivation. Human Genetics. 2011;**130**:307-327

[80] Kharbanda KK. Role of transmethylation reactions in alcoholic liver disease. World Journal of Gastroenterology. 2007;**13**:4947-4954

[81] Kriaucionis S, Heintz N. The nuclear DNA base 5-hydroxymethylcytosine is present in Purkinje neurons and the brain. Science. 2009;**324**:929-930

[82] Tahiliani M, Koh KP, Shen Y, Pastor WA, Bandukwala H, Brudno Y, et al. Conversion of 5-methylcytosine to 5-hydroxymethylcytosine in mammalian DNA by MLL partner TET1. Science. 2009;**324**:930-935

[83] Bhutani N, Burns DM, Blau HM. DNA demethylation dynamics. Cell. 2011;**146**:866-872

[84] Kohli RM, Zhang Y. TET enzymes, TDG and the dynamics of DNA demethylation. Nature. 2013;**502**: 472-479

[85] Ecsedi S, Rodríguez-Aguilera JR, Hernández-Vargas H. 5-Hydroxymethylcytosine (5hmC), or how to identify your favorite cell. Epigenomes. 2018;**2**(1):3

[86] Mellen M, Ayata P, Dewell S, Kriaucionis S, Heintz N. MeCP2 binds to 5hmC enriched within active genes and accessible chromatin in the nervous system. Cell. 2012;**151**:1417-1430

[87] Chagoya de Sanchez V, Hernandez-Munoz R, Sanchez L, Vidrio S, Yanez L, Suarez J. Twenty-four-hour changes of S-adenosylmethionine, S-adenosylhomocysteine adenosine and their metabolizing enzymes in rat liver; possible physiological significance in phospholipid methylation. The International Journal of Biochemistry. 1991;**23**:1439-1443

[88] Komatsu Y, Waku T, Iwasaki N, Ono W, Yamaguchi C, Yanagisawa J. Global analysis of DNA methylation in early-stage liver fibrosis. BMC Medical Genomics. 2012;**5**:5

[89] Page A, Paoli P, Moran Salvador E, White S, French J, Mann J. Hepatic stellate cell transdifferentiation involves genome-wide remodeling of the DNA methylation landscape. Journal of Hepatology. 2016;**64**:661-673

[90] Arenas-Huertero F, Recillas-Targa F. Chromatin epigenetic modifications in cancer generation. Gaceta Médica de México. 2002;**138**:547-555

[91] Valdes-Quezada C, Arriaga-Canon C, Fonseca-Guzman Y, Guerrero G, Recillas-Targa F. CTCF demarcates chicken embryonic alpha-globin gene autonomous silencing and contributes to adult stage-specific gene expression. Epigenetics. 2013;**8**:827-838

[92] Felsenfeld G, Groudine M. Controlling the double helix. Nature. 2003;**421**:448-453

[93] Yao W, Wang T, Huang F. p300/CBP as a key nutritional sensor for hepatic energy homeostasis and liver fibrosis. BioMed Research International. 2018;**2018**:8168791

[94] Mann J, Chu DC, Maxwell A, Oakley F, Zhu NL, Tsukamoto H, et al. MeCP2 controls an epigenetic pathway that promotes myofibroblast transdifferentiation and fibrosis. Gastroenterology. 2010;**138**:705, 714 e1-714, 714 e4

[95] Bosch FX, Ribes J, Cleries R, Diaz M. Epidemiology of hepatocellular carcinoma. Clinical Liver Disease. 2005; **9**:191-211

[96] The L. GLOBOCAN 2018: Counting the toll of cancer. Lancet. 2018;**392**:985

[97] Marquardt JU, Seo D, Andersen JB, Gillen MC, Kim MS, Conner EA, et al. Sequential transcriptome analysis of

human liver cancer indicates late stage acquisition of malignant traits. Journal of Hepatology. 2014;**60**:346-353

[98] Castelli G, Pelosi E, Testa U. Liver cancer: Molecular characterization, clonal evolution and cancer stem cells. Cancers (Basel). 2017;**9**(9):127

[99] Miyata T, Yamashita YI, Baba Y, Harada K, Yamao T, Umezaki N, et al. Prognostic value of LINE-1 methylation level in 321 patients with primary liver cancer including hepatocellular carcinoma and intrahepatic cholangiocarcinoma. Oncotarget. 2018; **9**:20795-20806

[100] Fan G, Tu Y, Chen C, Sun H, Wan C, Cai X. DNA methylation biomarkers for hepatocellular carcinoma. Cancer Cell International. 2018;**18**:140

[101] Yang H, Liu Y, Bai F, Zhang JY, Ma SH, Liu J, et al. Tumor development is associated with decrease of TET gene expression and 5-methylcytosine hydroxylation. Oncogene. 2013;**32**: 663-669

[102] Li X, Liu Y, Salz T, Hansen KD, Feinberg A. Whole-genome analysis of the methylome and hydroxymethylome in normal and malignant lung and liver. Genome Research. 2016;**26**:1730-1741

[103] Dimitroulis D, Damaskos C, Valsami S, Davakis S, Garmpis N, Spartalis E, et al. From diagnosis to treatment of hepatocellular carcinoma: An epidemic problem for both developed and developing world. World Journal of Gastroenterology. 2017;**23**: 5282-5294

[104] Llovet JM, Schwartz M, Mazzaferro V. Resection and liver transplantation for hepatocellular carcinoma. Seminars in Liver Disease. 2005;**25**:181-200

[105] Nguyen K, Jack K, Sun W. Hepatocellular carcinoma: Past and future of molecular target therapy. Diseases. 2015;**4**(1):1

[106] Deng GL, Zeng S, Shen H. Chemotherapy and target therapy for hepatocellular carcinoma: New advances and challenges. World Journal of Hepatology. 2015;**7**:787-798

[107] Khemlina G, Ikeda S, Kurzrock R. The biology of hepatocellular carcinoma: Implications for genomic and immune therapies. Molecuar Cancer. 2017;**16**:149

[108] Sanoff HK, Chang Y, Lund JL, O'Neil BH, Dusetzina SB. Sorafenib effectiveness in advanced hepatocellular carcinoma. The Oncologist. 2016;**21**: 1113-1120

[109] Velasco-Loyden G, Perez-Martinez L, Vidrio-Gomez S, Perez-Carreon JI, Chagoya de Sanchez V. Cancer chemoprevention by an adenosine derivative in a model of cirrhosis-hepatocellular carcinoma induced by diethylnitrosamine in rats. Tumour Biology. 2017;**39**:1010428317691190

[110] Chavez E, Lozano-Rosas MG, Dominguez-Lopez M, Velasco-Loyden G, Rodriguez-Aguilera JR, Jose-Nunez C, et al. Functional, metabolic, and dynamic mitochondrial changes in the rat cirrhosis-hepatocellular carcinoma model and the protective effect of IFC-305. Journal of Pharmacology and Experimental Therapeutics. 2017;**361** (2):292-302

Chapter 7

Nonischemic Cardiomyopathy in Liver Transplant Recipients

Alexander A. Vitin, Dana Tomescu and Leonard Azamfirei

Abstract

Nonischemic cardiomyopathy is a collective term, encompassing a spectrum of cardiac comorbidities, accompanying the progressing end-stage liver disease. Alcoholic and cirrhotic cardiomyopathies are the most researched, well-known clinical entities in the list of nonischemic cardiac disorders that bear the most substantial impact on the clinical course, management, and outcomes of liver transplantation in ESLD patients. In this chapter, morphology, pathophysiology, diagnostic criteria, clinical manifestations, and management options of nonischemic cardiomyopathy in liver transplant candidates and recipients, the patients with end-stage liver disease due to advanced stages of cirrhosis, are discussed.

Keywords: nonischemic cardiomyopathy, cirrhosis, liver transplantation, morphology, physiology, management

1. Introduction

The trend of performing liver transplants on an ever-increasing number of sicker patients with more severe cardio-vascular comorbidities, once considered as posing insurmountably high risk, prohibitive for surgery, is quickly becoming an everyday reality. Among other comorbidities, cardiomyopathies are considered as very common conditions that significantly alter the course of the liver disease and candidacy for liver transplant and contributes substantially to perioperative hemodynamic profile and management and, eventually, to immediate and long-term outcome. While coronary artery disease-related morbidity remains the most serious concern in respect to liver transplant recipient well-being and outcomes, the groups of nonischemic cardiac conditions, that are increasingly common, oftentimes go underappreciated, underdiagnosed, and simply overlooked. The recent trends, however, demonstrate an increasing awareness and deeper understanding of these conditions.

Limited data is available about the actual prevalence of cardiomyopathy and its impact on the liver transplantation outcome. According to recent studies, it has been estimated that as many as 50% of patients undergoing liver transplantation developed at least some signs of cardiac dysfunction [1], and overall mortality from overt heart failure in the post liver transplantation period was estimated at about 7–21% [2].

In this review, we will focus on physiological and clinical aspects of nonischemic cardiomyopathy, which accompany practically every liver disease in the advanced stages.

Nowadays, the majority of transplant subspecialty physicians consider cardiomyopathy mostly as either "cirrhotic" or "alcoholic," with disregard to differences in physiology, clinical course and, for liver transplant recipients, even to outcome impact.

We suggest considering a "cardiomyopathy" as a collective term that refers to the spectrum of myocardial pathology, with a variety of etiological factors, ways and timing of development, similar, albeit not exactly identical, clinical manifestations, and degrees of contribution to hemodynamic profile of the liver transplant recipient. Furthermore, based on clinical features, cardiac morbidities, encountered in liver transplant candidates/recipients that qualify for nonischemic cardiomyopathy, may be divided into chronic forms (such as cirrhotic, alcoholic, etc.) and acute (stress-induced and Takotsubo).

In this review, we will focus on etiology, morphology, pathophysiology, diagnostic criteria, and clinical manifestations of chronic nonischemic cardiomyopathies in liver transplant candidates. Acute nonischemic stress-induced cardiomyopathy discussion is beyond this chapter's scope.

2. Etiology-related morphology

Etiologically different forms of cardiomyopathy have generally similar pathological morphology and histopathology, with minimal, sometimes imperceptible, differences in microscopic details. In majority of cases, a histomorphological picture of nonischemic cardiomyopathy may be identified as having common features with chronic myocarditis, resulting in myocardial fibrosis, hypertrophic, dilated cardiomyopathy, or their combination.

As it has been demonstrated (using endomyocardial biopsy), a distinction between idiopathic, chronic inflammatory, and alcoholic cardiomyopathy is virtually impossible. Common features such as fibrosis, cardiac myocyte hypertrophy, and nuclear alterations have been observed in the alcoholic cardiomyopathy [3] or the World Heart Federation/International Society and Federation of Cardiomyopathy (WHF/ISFC) definition of myocarditis [4, 5]. Alcohol consumption is considered to be the major contributory factor of secondary nonischemic dilated cardiomyopathy in up to 33% of all cases of dilated cardiomyopathy [6, 7]. In alcoholic cardiomyopathy, dilation and impaired contraction of the left or both ventricles are observed [8]. Left ventricular end-diastolic diameters are increased compared to age- and weight-matched controls, the left ventricular mass index is increased, and the left ventricular ejection fraction is well below normal (<45%) [9].

Recent studies have demonstrated that Hepatitis C virus (HCV) also possesses tropism trait for other than liver tissues, such as lymphatic system and myocardial cell membranes. However, precise mechanisms of the myocardial damage have not yet been elucidated. Development of HCV-associated cardiomyopathy is considered as a result of multiple factors, such as viral, immunologic, and apoptotic-related in genetically susceptible patients [10]. Recent studies have demonstrated hepatitis C virus (HCV) involvement in the development of dilated cardiomyopathy, hypertrophic cardiomyopathy, and arrhythmogenic right ventricular cardiomyopathy in addition to myocarditis and myocardial fibrosis [11].

Cirrhotic cardiomyopathy is defined as "cardiac dysfunction in patients with cirrhosis, characterized by impaired contractile responsiveness to stress, diastolic dysfunction, and electrophysiological abnormalities in the absence of known cardiac disease" [12]. There is only very limited information about epidemiology, as well as actual prevalence of this condition at present time. Its diagnosis is difficult, because the majority of liver transplant candidates demonstrate nearly normal (for cirrhotic patient) cardiac function at rest, and only during ESLD decompensation phases, they present with diastolic and/or high cardiac output heart failure [13]. However, QT interval prolongation in cirrhotic patients (25% in cirrhosis Child Pugh class A, 51% in Child Pugh class B, and 60% in Child Pugh class C) may be considered the earliest sign of cirrhotic cardiomyopathy; some information of prevalence might be derived from these data [14–16]. In earlier studies, cirrhotic cardiomyopathy has been considered to be related to both portal hypertension and cirrhosis itself, and is characterized by intrinsic alterations in myocardial function [17]. In its advanced stages, the morphology of cirrhotic cardiomyopathy may be described as, essentially, a combination of both dilated and hypertrophic cardiomyopathy, with various degrees of fibrosis development. Oftentimes, right- or bilateral atrial enlargement, along with right ventricle distension may be seen using TTE.

Hemochromatosis, due to iron deposition in myocardial cells, predisposes to either dilated or restrictive cardiomyopathy. If left untreated, hemochromatosis eventually progresses to end-stage heart and liver disease, with heart-liver transplantation as the best treatment option [18]. Early electrocardiographic abnormalities are frequent in patients with cirrhosis due to hemochromatosis. However, overt CHF is unusual [19]. Morphology of hemochromatosis-related cardiomyopathy in cirrhotic patients includes increased left ventricular mass, end-diastolic and end-systolic diameters of the left ventricle, and left atrium diameters, as well as significant changes of systolic function indices [20].

Nonalcoholic fat liver disease is becoming highly prevalent in the adult population (15–30%), with increase to 70–90% in obesity and type 2 diabetes, representing one of the most common causes of chronic liver disease among LT candidates [21, 22]. The correlation between almost two-fold increased cardiovascular mortality and nonalcoholic steatohepatitis (NASH) has been clearly demonstrated [23]. Increased amounts of liver fat are associated with the presence of markers of inflammation and risk factors of coronary vascular disease, independent of BMI. Steatosis has been found to be the strongest independent risk predictor of vascular damage and also involved in pathogenesis of coronary vascular disease in liver transplant candidates. In a recent study, severe early LV diastolic and systolic dysfunctions were observed in NASH patients [24–26]. In a retrospective study, comparing patients with nonalcoholic steatohepatitis (NASH) and alcoholic cirrhosis, NASH was more frequently associated with cardiovascular events after liver transplant in comparison with that in the alcoholic cirrhotic patients [27, 28]. Although coronary artery disease and related ischemic cardiomyopathy is beyond the scope of this review, it seems worth mentioning the involvement of such common etiology of ESLD, such as NASH cirrhosis, in cardiomyopathy development.

3. Pathophysiology and mechanisms of nonischemic cardiomyopathy

3.1 Contractility impairment, systolic dysfunction, and diastolic dysfunction

Overall myocardial dysfunction physiology in cirrhotic patients is exceedingly complex, multicomponent, and still not entirely understood. Two main components should be considered: myocardial contractility impairment and contribution of high cardiac output & low afterload hemodynamic profile (typical for ESLD patient hyperdynamic circulation), with secondary hemodynamic derangements, such as portopulmonary hypertension and related syndromes.

In their comprehensive review, Møller and Hendriksen [12] listed a number of potential mechanisms involved in the impairment of contractile function of the cardiomyocyte in cirrhotic cardiomyopathy on the receptor level. These include:

downregulation of b-adrenergic receptors with decreased content of G-protein, causing inotropic incompetency, and upregulation of cannabinoid 1-receptor stimulation; increased inhibitory effects of cardiodepressant substances such as hemoxygenase, carbon monoxide (CO), nitric oxide synthase (NOS)-induced nitric oxide (NO) release, and tumor necrosis factor-α(TNF – α). Many postreceptor effects are mediated by adenylyl cyclase inhibition or stimulation. Altered function and reduced conductance of potassium channels, inhibition of L-type calcium channels, and increased fluidity of the plasma membrane (increased cholesterol/phospholipid ratio) also contribute to reduced calcium release and contractility.

It has been demonstrated that the reduced β - adrenergetic-dependent inotropic effect could be attributed to an overexpression of inhibitory G-protein and regulators of G-protein signaling, which inhibit the adenylate cyclase, and those that accelerate degradation of cAMP such as phosphodiesterase [29]. The endogenous and exogenous cannabinoids exert mostly a vasodilatory effect. The ability of endocannabinoids to induce apoptosis of hepatic stellate cells, promoting the development of portal hypertension and hyperdynamic circulation, amplifies by vasodilation [30]. Increased local endocannabinoid production in cirrhosis and activation of CB1 receptors by endogenous anandamide contributes to the reduced cardiac contractility in cirrhosis [31].

Experimental evidence suggests that nitric oxide (NO) plays a significant role in the decreased vascular responsiveness to vasoconstrictors [32]. NO has been shown to cause significant impairment of the contractility in cirrhotic rats. Results of experimental studies have indicated that the cytokine–NO pathway occurs in cirrhotic rat hearts with enhanced expression of the NO synthase, and that inhibition of the NO synthesis by the NO inhibitor L-NAME reverses the impaired cardiac contractility [33–35].

Abnormalities in the properties of the plasma membrane determine the magnitude of the ion channel dysfunction. A decreased density of potassium currents in ventricular myocytes, which may contribute to prolong the QT interval, has been found on an experimental model. Also, a reduced expression and density of L-type Ca++ channels and inward cellular calcium current have been found as well, which may contribute to reduced contractility and also cause changes in excitation-contraction coupling and prolonged QT interval, with arrhythmogenic effect ensued [36–38].

B-type natriuretic peptide (BNP) and its prohormone, pro-BNP, are sensitive markers of even mild myocardial injury. Both compounds have been found elevated in patients with compensated and decompensated cirrhosis and seemingly correlate with the severity of cardiac dysfunction and myocardial hypertrophy [39, 40].

All aforementioned mechanisms of contractility impairment contribute to systolic dysfunction development. In majority of liver transplant candidates, the left ventricular ejection fraction (LVEF), which serves as relatively integral index of systolic function assessment, has been found normal (EF of 50–60%) or increased (EF > 70%) at rest in patients with cirrhosis [41, 42]. Some attenuation of LVEF has been shown after exercise, sodium load, or erect posture [43]. Blunted heart rate response to stress, reduced myocardial reserve, and impaired muscular oxygen extraction are among reasons that potentially contribute to the systolic dysfunction in cirrhotic patients [44].

Diastolic dysfunction is characterized by abnormal left ventricular relaxation, impeding blood flow through the ventricle, increasing left ventricular end-diastolic pressure, and increasing atrial contribution to late ventricular filling [45]. Diastolic dysfunction may be a consequence of either hypertrophic or dilated cardiomyopathy, myocardial patchy fibrosis, and subendothelial edema [46]. The histopathology of diastolic dysfunction showed cardiomyocyte hypertrophy, altered pigmentation, interstitial fibrosis, and myofiber vacuolization [47]. Diastolic dysfunction, manifesting in impaired passive and active filling of the left ventricle during diastole, causes an inability to adequately increase stroke volume in response to stress and other stimuli. Diastolic dysfunction may precede systolic dysfunction in cirrhosis [48]. The clinical significance of diastolic dysfunction has been best demonstrated in cases of rapidly developing heart failure after transjugular intrahepatic portosystemic shunts (TIPS) [49]. It has been found that after TIPS, there is an increase in the left atrial diameter, the pulmonary capillary wedge pressure, and total pulmonary resistance [50].

3.2 Role of the hyperdynamic circulation

As it has been shown in numerous studies, peripheral and splanchnic vasodilatation appears to be the leading cause of hyperdynamic circulation in advanced stages of ESLD [51]. Initially, a reduction in systemic vascular resistance is compensated by an increase in cardiac output (almost to 200% of baseline), and effective circulating blood volume satisfies the requirements for adequate peripheral perfusion. In advanced stages of cirrhosis, a further reduction in systemic vascular resistance cannot be compensated by a further increase in cardiac output, which leads to relative "hypovolemia" that manifests in hemodynamic instability and poor stress (e.g. blood loss) tolerance. At this stage, other mechanisms, such as activation of the renin-angiotensin system, sympathetic nervous system, and antidiuretic hormone overproduction, are employed to maintain effective circulating blood volume and perfusion pressure. Activation of these same compensatory systems is the leading cause of sodium and water retention and, ultimately, ascites formation [52, 53].

Though overt heart failure in even advanced stages of ESLD is a rare occurrence, the compensation mechanisms eventually are becoming overwhelmed, and, in a view of very limited myocardial reserve, already impaired contractility, systolic and diastolic dysfunctions, and myocardial performance are starting to decline substantially.

3.3 Role of portopulmonary hypertension

Portopulmonary hypertension is defined as pulmonary hypertension, associated with portal hypertension with or without accompanying liver cirrhosis. The correlation between development of portopulmonary hypertension and the severity of liver disease has not been found. Approximately 20% of candidates for liver transplantation will have elevated pulmonary artery pressures, but have a normal pulmonary vascular resistance (PVR). Such PA pressure increase may be the result of volume overload, cardiac failure, and high output circulation. True portopulmonary hypertension has a prevalence of 5–6% among liver transplant candidates and is the result of pathological changes in the pulmonary vasculature [54].

In the assessment of a liver transplant candidate, presenting with portopulmonary hypertension, a right heart catheterization, a transthoracic echocardiography, and a test-challenge with volume bolus and dobutamine test are instrumental in determining the limits of patient's tolerance for potential liver transplantation procedure [55].

The most important component of the porto-pulmonary syndrome physiology is, actually, not so much the degree of pulmonary hypertension, expressed in pulmonary artery pressure figures, but rather right ventricle (RV) dysfunction, namely significant shape (i.e. RV dilation) and systolic function alterations. In the group of patients with more rapid increase in PAP (as opposed to the slow, gradual pulmonary hypertension development), early RV dilation and more significant pulmonary regurgitation, leading to various degrees of right ventricular failure and decompensation, have been found [56].

Portopulmonary hypertension has an enormous impact on liver transplantation outcome. A mean pulmonary artery pressure (MPAP) of 50 mm Hg or greater has been found to be associated with a 100% post-OLT mortality rate, and a MPAP of 35 to <50 mm Hg is associated with a 50% post-OLT mortality rate [57]. For the time being, severe portopulmonary hypertension is considered to be an absolute contra-indication to liver transplant. Patients with moderate severity should be considered for pulmonary vasodilator therapy, and their candidacy for liver transplantation depends on their hemodynamic response [58].

Liver transplantation may not reverse the portopulmonary hypertension. Long-term vasodilator therapy may be necessary after the surgery, and, nevertheless, the syndrome may persist for years [59, 60].

It remains unclear, to which exact degree portopulmonary hypertension contributes to worsening of preexisting cardiomyopathy. However, its role in the development of right ventricle dilation and ultimate right heart failure appears to be more significant than commonly recognized.

4. Diagnostic criteria

A proposal for diagnostic and supportive criteria for cirrhotic cardiomyopathy agreed upon at the 2005 World Congress of Gastroenterology in Montreal published in 2008, a working definition of cirrhotic cardiomyopathy is formulated as follows: "A cardiac dysfunction in patients with cirrhosis characterized by impaired contractile responsiveness to stress and/or altered diastolic relaxation with electrophysiological abnormalities in the absence of other known cardiac diseases." The diagnostic criteria are summarized in **Table 1**.

While systolic dysfunction ECO-diagnosis is more or less straightforward, diastolic dysfunction sometimes presents a certain challenge. TTE/TEE diagnostic criteria of diastolic dysfunction include decreased ratio of early to late atrial phases of ventricular filling (E/A ratio, less than 1). The decreased E/A ratio is a relatively common finding in cirrhotic patients [43, 61]. Measurement of the mitral annular E

Systolic dysfunction
1. Blunted increase in cardiac output on exercise, volume challenge, or pharmacological stimuli 2. Resting ejection fraction, 55%
Diastolic dysfunction
1. E/A ratio, 1.0 (age-corrected) 2. Prolonged deceleration time (0.200 ms)
Supportive criteria
1. Electrophysiological abnormalities: • Abnormal chronotropic response • Electromechanical uncoupling/dyssynchrony • Prolonged Q–Tc interval 2. Enlarged left atrium 3. Increased myocardial mass 4. Increased BNP and pro-BNP 5. Increased troponin I
BNP, brain natriuretic peptide; E/A ratio, ratio of early to late (atrial) phases of ventricular filling (from: 46, with modifications).

Table 1.
Diagnostic criteria of cirrhotic cardiomyopathy.

wave (E′) is considered a more accurate marker for evaluation of diastolic dysfunction, due to its decreased dependency on the preload in the presence of diastolic dysfunction. With worsening of the diastolic dysfunction, the E′ decreases, which reflects the increased stiffness of the ventricle. The E:E′ ratio has been found to reflect left ventricular filling pressure, and this ratio increases as diastolic function worsens [62–65].

5. Clinical manifestations and reversibility

The clinical manifestations of cirrhosis-related myocardial dysfunction are becoming evident during liver transplantation surgery, when the hemodynamics are affected by numerous factors that include blood loss and fluid shifts with substantial third space formation, mechanical ventilation, large vessel clamping (specifically portal vein and IVC), and effects of anesthesia. In severe cases, heart failure manifests in significant reduction in the cardiac output [66, 67]. The problem is that, considering the baseline abnormally increased CO (up to 10–12 L/min), a gradual decrease to 4–5 L/min may not be immediately perceived as such and interpreted as a sign of ongoing myocardial decompensation. In the clinical study on 209 liver transplant recipients, abnormal cardiac response was observed in 47 (22.5%) patients after reperfusion. The authors suggested that the abnormal cardiac response observed during liver transplantation is a manifestation of occult cirrhotic cardiomyopathy [68].

A number of factors affect myocardial performance in the immediate postoperative period. Persisting metabolic disturbances, specifically lactic acidosis, hypothermia, and electrolyte disturbances (hyperkalemia and hypocalcemia) can further compromise cardiac performance. Among multiple causes of postoperative hemodynamic instability (such as underestimated hypovolemia due to ongoing or occult hemorrhage, third space formation/losses), a preexisting dilated cardiomyopathy should not be overlooked.

The rapid improvement of systemic vasodilatation, especially in combination with use of vasoactive agents, can result in a sudden increase in the afterload, which is another possible cause of excessive myocardial stress, leading to potential development or worsening of the existing heart failure. It has been found that after liver transplantation, almost 25% of liver transplant recipients have cardiovascular complications and an increased risk for postoperative pulmonary edema [16]. Postoperative pulmonary edema is quite common occurrence, and at least 50% of edema episodes develop within the first 24 h after surgery [69].

Reversibility of cardiomyopathy after liver transplant, albeit previously presumed very likely, appears to be not all that assured, let alone guaranteed, according to recent clinical studies. In the retrospective study on 243 liver transplant recipients, the diastolic dysfunction and QT interval changes have been investigated in postoperative period. The results revealed that the grade of diastolic dysfunction significantly worsened on echo performed after transplantation. Diastolic function worsened in up to 40% of the patients. Furthermore, longer QT was independently associated with adverse outcomes after OLT. Although QT significantly decreased after OLT, prolonged QT continued to be prevalent among patients after OLT. However, as study demonstrated that despite being associated with a longer hospital stay, the presence of diastolic dysfunction was not independently associated with long-term adverse outcomes after OLT. The authors concluded that some parameters, representing cirrhotic cardiomyopathy, such as diastolic dysfunction and prolongation of QT, continued to worsen or, at least persist in patients for many years after OLT [70].

6. Management: possible treatment options

Universally accepted treatment for clinically significant cardiomyopathy is yet to be established. Pharmacological interventions should be directed at the most important components of the syndrome, such as systolic and diastolic dysfunction, electrophysiological abnormalities, and impaired contractility. Liver transplant remains an ultimate cure for cirrhosis and for its major complications; it is also likely to cure the cirrhotic cardiomyopathy. However, neither time frame nor the extent of myocardial functional and structural recovery is known yet.

Nonselective β-blockers have been shown to improve the prolonged QT interval; β-blockers-induced cardiac output modification/reduction might play a positive role in the reduction of the hyperdynamic load [71, 72].

The common principles of the congestive heart failure treatment are completely applicable and should be followed, once heart failure manifests in liver transplant recipient. Depending on renal function (or lack thereof, in cases of severe hepatorenal syndrome or acute kidney injury), the treatment of CHF in cirrhotic patient will, most likely, include diuretics. It is likely, that patients with manifesting heart failure also exhibit a diuretic-resistant ascites. Even in these cases, aldosterone antagonists, such as spironolactone, might be beneficial in reducing left ventricular hypertrophy and dilatation, potentially improving diastolic dysfunction [73]. The known effects of aldosterone, such as myocardial fibrosis development, and baroreceptor dysfunction, provide a rationale for using an aldosterone antagonist, to counteract these effects [74].

The most significant hemodynamic instability, occurring during liver transplantation surgery, may be partially attributed, among other well-recognized factors (such as inherently low Systemic Vascular Resistance (SVR), to the manifestation or exacerbation of myocardial dysfunction due to preexiting cardiomyopathy.

At the start of the anhepatic stage, the portal cross clamp causes a variable (20–30% of baseline) degree of venous return decrease. IVC complete cross-clamp oftentimes leads to a more substantial and poorer tolerated (approximately 50%) decrease of venous return, whereas IVC partial clamp causes a variable, about 25–50%, decrease of venous return [75]. This rapid decrease in preload may be tolerated poorly by patients with ESLD. These patients have notoriously very limited ability, if any, to compensate for the rapid decrease in venous return with systemic vasoconstriction, due to inherent low SVR.

The possible solution to compensate, at least temporarily, for the decreased venous return (thus drop in cardiac output, which becomes substantially more pronounced in patients with both systolic and diastolic dysfunctions) is a venovenous bypass (VVB). It has been suggested that hypotension (30% decrease in MAP) or a decrease in cardiac index (50%) during a 5-min test period of hepatic vascular occlusion can be used to identify the group of patients, who require VVB. Other indications to the VVB include the presence of pulmonary hypertension, impaired ventricular function from previous myocardial infarction, ischemic heart disease, and cardiomyopathy [76, 77].

In patients with pulmonary hypertension (either idiopathic or due to portpulmonary syndrome), excessive fluid loading to compensate for hypovolemia-related hemodynamic instability may result in acute right ventricular dysfunction. Patients with preexisting cardiomyopathy, mostly impaired left ventricular function, express a limited ability to generate an adequate CO. These patients, too, may benefit from the ameliorative effect of the preload, associated with VVB, throughout the whole of liver transplant surgery, but particularly during anhepatic and postreperfusion stages [67].

In the view of rapid hemodynamic changes, associated with IVC either complete or even partial clamps, large amounts of fluids, along with blood products, are often needed to be administered. In patients with impaired renal function (ranging from acute kidney injury to hepatorenal syndrome and end-stage renal disease, intraoperative dialysis is used, mostly for the purposes of renal function complete replacement or preservation. Hemodialysis is also very efficient means of intravascular volume regulation, specifically in elimination of fluid overload [78]. These properties make hemodialysis and hemofiltration valuable and efficient tools also in decreasing a burden on dysfunctional myocardium, particularly in patients with substantial diastolic dysfunction due to cardiomyopathy. The target is to achieve euvolemia or a zero balance ultrafiltration volume by the use of hemodialysis, which becomes especially beneficial after IVC unclamping, the very intraoperative event, that causes notoriously substantial right ventricle volume overload, with potential to decompensation in cases of advanced cardiomyopathy [79].

Graft reperfusion and postreperfusion syndrome presents the most significant challenge for hemodynamic management, especially in patients with severe cardiomyopathy. Different drug combinations have been tested and recommended for rapid hemodynamic recovery after liver graft reperfusion. Vasopressin in small boluses, 1–2 U, may be highly efficient in opposing the significant and rapid decrease of SVR, and calcium chloride, up to 1000 mg, may enhance inotropic effects of epinephrine [67, 80]. Methylene blue, 2 mg/kg, has been reported as very efficient and "last resort" drug for prolong and profound hypotension, refractory to treatment with other vasoactive drugs [81]. The immediate hemodynamic stabilization (on the face of severely compromised myocardial function, in combination with rapid decrease in SVR, observed during postreperfusion stage), which all these drug combinations provide, should be further maintained with continuous infusion administration of vasoactive agents, such as phenylephrine or vasopressin, targeting primarily reduction of systemic vascular resistance. Compromised myocardial performance due to preexisting dilated cardiomyopathy and especially its worsening after graft reperfusion oftentimes necessitates addition of agents with β-adrenergic activities, such as norepinephrine, and, rarely, epinephrine [82, 83].

To better understand the causes and mechanisms of blunted cardiac response to stress and inotropic incompetence, investigations on the gene expression pattern of the cardiomyocyte adrenergic pathway in animal models of cirrhosis are underway [84]. New gene-targeting pharmacological strategies, based on the findings of these studies, might be the future direction of the cardiomyopathy treatment, and also, of course, a promising new direction of the research.

The normalization of cardiac function after liver transplantation is still a likely and attainable goal in majority of cases, provided all treatment modalities are employed in full and timely manner, and, above all, the liver transplantation procedure is successful.

7. Conclusions

The term "nonischemic cardiomyopathy" represents a spectrum of cardiac comorbidities, encountered in the liver transplant recipient at every stage of the process, namely, in preoperative period, intraoperatively, and during recovery. Alcoholic and cirrhotic cardiomyopathies are the well-known clinical entities. Yet, oftentimes, these conditions remain unrecognized and underdiagnosed in clinical setting.

Morphology of nonischemic cardiomyopathy includes various anatomical derangements, ranging from right and/or left atrial enlargement/distention to severe ventricular dilation and constrictive changes, with correspondent profound physiological effects that include significant diastolic, followed by systolic, dysfunction and eventually resulting in the frank heart failure. Rhythm disturbances are very common, and serve as an early diagnostic sign of the developing cardiomyopathy.

To date, a consensus on causes, physiological mechanisms, and, most importantly, management and treatment of nonischemic cardiomyopathy is yet to be achieved. The existing management and treatment modalities are directed mostly on hemodynamic optimization at every stage of the transplantation process, and remain extremely complex and challenging intraoperatively, when a clinician faces multilevel surgery-related hemodynamic derangements, exacerbated greatly by the presence of clinically significant cardiomyopathy.

Decades of experience has shown that at least complete hemodynamic recovery, if not a meaningful structural and functional restoration of the myocardium, is an achievable goal in liver transplant recipients, and recent studies in this particular field have achieved promising results.

Further research on physiology, genetics, and treatment options is warranted, and results of multicenter studies, involving large numbers of liver transplant recipients, are much needed to be implemented to ensure successful outcome of liver transplantation in recipients, suffering from nonischemic cardiomyopathy.

Author details

Alexander A. Vitin[1*], Dana Tomescu[2] and Leonard Azamfirei[3]

1 Department of Anesthesiology, University of Washington, Seattle, WA, USA

2 Department of Anesthesia and Intensive Care, Fundeni Clinical Institute, “Carol Davila” University of Medicine and Pharmacy, Bucharest, Romania

3 University of Medicine and Pharmacy Tîrgu Mureş, Tîrgu Mureş, Romania

*Address all correspondence to: vitin@uw.edu

References

[1] Myers RP, Lee SS. Cirrhotic cardiomyopathy and liver transplantation. Liver Transplantation. Jul 2000;**6**(4 Suppl 1):S44-S52

[2] Baik SK, Fouad TR, Lee SS. Cirrhotic cardiomyopathy. Orphanet Journal of Rare Diseases. 2007;**2**:15-23

[3] Teragaki M, Takeuchi K, Takeda T. Clinical and histologic features of alcohol drinkers with congestive heart failure. American Heart Journal. 1993;**125**:808-817

[4] Maisch B, Portic I, Ristic AD. Definition of inflammatory cardiomyopathy (myocarditis): On the way to consensus. Herz. 2000;**25**(3):200-209

[5] Maisch B. Alcoholic cardiomyopathy. Herz. 2016;**41**:484-493. DOI: 10.1007/s00059-016-4469-6

[6] Rubin E, Urbano-Marquez A. Alcoholic cardiomyopathy. Alcoholism, Clinical and Experimental Research. 1994;**18**:111-114

[7] Piano MR, Schwertz DW. Alcoholic heart disease: A review. Heart & Lung. 1994;**23**:3-17

[8] Preedy VR, Atkinson LM, Richardson PJ, Peters TJ. Mechanisms of ethanol-induced cardiac damage. British Heart Journal. 1994;**69**:197-200

[9] Kupari M, Koskinen P, Suokas A. Left ventricular size, mass and function in relation to the duration and quantity of heavy drinking in alcoholics. The American Journal of Cardiology. 1991;**67**:274-279

[10] Sanchez MJ, Bergasa NV. Hepatitis C associated cardiomyopathy: Potential pathogenic mechanisms and clinical implications. Medical Science Monitor. 2008;**14**(5):RA55-RA63

[11] Matsumori A. Role of hepatitis C virus in cardiomyopathies. Ernst Schering Research Foundation Workshop. 2006;**55**:99-120

[12] Møller S, Henriksen JH. Cirrhotic cardiomyopathy. Journal of Hepatology. 2010;**53**:179-190

[13] Zardi EM, Abbate A, Zardi DM, Dobrina A, Margiotta D, et al. Cirrhotic cardiomyopathy. Journal of the American College of Cardiology. 2010;**56**:539-549

[14] Fede G, Privitera G, Tomaselli T, Spadaro L, Purrello F. Cardiovascular dysfunction in patients with liver cirrhosis. Annals of Gastroenterology. 2015;**28**:31-40

[15] Bernardi M, Maggioli C, Dibra V, Zaccherini G. QT interval prolongation in liver cirrhosis: Innocent bystander or serious threat? Expert Review of Gastroenterology & Hepatology. 2012;**6**:57-66

[16] Zardi EM, Zardi DM, Chin D, Sonnino C, Dobrina A, et al. Cirrhotic cardiomyopathy in the pre- and post-liver transplantation phase. Journal of Cardiology. 2016;**67**:125-130

[17] Donovan CL, Marcovitz PA, Punch JD, Bach DS, Brown KA, Lucey MR. Two dimensional and dobutamine stress echocardiography in the preoperative assessment of patients with end-stage liver disease prior to orthotopic liver transplantation. Transplantation. 1996;**61**:1180-1188

[18] Kremastinos DT, Farmakis D. Iron overload cardiomyopathy in clinical practice. Circulation. 2011;**124**:2253-2263

[19] Niederau C, Fischer R, Purschel A, Stremmel W, Haussinger D, Strohmeyer G. Long-term survival in patients

with hereditary hemochromatosis. Gastroenterology. 1996;**110**:1107-1119

[20] Shizukuda Y, Bolan CD, Tripodi DJ, Yau YY, Nguyen TT, Botello G, et al. Significance of left atrial contractile function in asymptomatic subjects with hereditary hemochromatosis. The American Journal of Cardiology. 2006;**98**:954-959

[21] Oni ET, Agatston AS, Blaha MJ, et al. A systematic review: Burden and severity of subclinical cardiovascular disease among those with nonalcoholic fatty liver; should we care? Atherosclerosis. 2013;**230**:258-267

[22] Kantartzis K, Stefan N. Cardiovascular disease in patients with non-alcoholic fatty liver disease. Annals of Gastroenterology. 2012;**25**:276-277

[23] Fouad YM, Yehia R. Hepato-cardiac disorders. World Journal of Hepatology. 2014;**6**(1):41-54

[24] Treeprasertsuk S, Lopez-Jimenez F, Lindor KD. Nonalcoholic fatty liver disease and the coronary artery disease. Digestive Diseases and Sciences. 2011;**56**:35-45

[25] Perseghin G. The role of non-alcoholic fatty liver disease in cardiovascular disease. Digestive Diseases. 2010;**28**:210-213

[26] Pacifico L, Di Martino M, De Merulis A, Bezzi M, Osborn JF, Catalano C, et al. Left ventricular dysfunction in obese children and adolescents with nonalcoholic fatty liver disease. Hepatology. Feb 2014;**59**(2):461-470. DOI: 10.1002/hep.26610. Epub 2013 Dec 23

[27] Targher G, Arcaro G. Non-alcoholic fatty liver disease and increased risk of cardiovascular disease. Atherosclerosis. 2007;**191**:235-240

[28] Vanwagner LB, Bhave M, Te HS, Feinglass J, Alvarez L, Rinella ME. Patients transplanted for nonalcoholic steatohepatitis are at increased risk for postoperative cardiovascular events. Hepatology. 2012;**56**:1741-1750

[29] Ceolotto G, Papparella I, Sticca A, Bova S, Cavalli M, Cargnelli G, et al. Anabnormal gene expression of the beta-adrenergic system contributes to the pathogenesis of cardiomyopathy in cirrhotic rats. Hepatology. 2008;**48**:1913-1923

[30] Moezi L, Gaskari SA, Lee SS. Endocannabinoids and liver disease. V. Endocannabinoids as mediators of vascular and cardiac abnormalities in cirrhosis. American Journal of Physiology-Gastrointestinal and Liver Physiology. 2008;**295**:G649-G653

[31] Gaskari SA, Liu H, Moezi L, Li Y, Baik SK, Lee SS. Role of endocannabinoids in the pathogenesis of cirrhotic cardiomyopathy in bile duct-ligated rats. British Journal of Pharmacology. 2005;**146**:315-323

[32] Castro A, Jimenez W, Claria J, Ros J, Martinez JM, Bosch M, et al. Impaired responsiveness to angiotensin-II in experimental cirrhosis–role of nitric oxide. Hepatology. 1993;**18**:367-372

[33] Van Obbergh L, Vallieres Y, Blaise G. Cardiac modifications occurring in the ascitic rat with biliary cirrhosis are nitric oxide related. Journal of Hepatology. 1996;**24**:747-752

[34] Garcia-Estan J, Ortiz MC, Lee SS. Nitric oxide and renal and cardiac dysfunction in cirrhosis. Clinical Science (London, England). 2002;**102**:213-222

[35] Liu H, Ma Z, Lee SS. Contribution of nitric oxide to the pathogenesis of cirrhotic cardiomyopathy in bile duct-ligated rats. Gastroenterology. 2000;**118**:937-944

[36] Ward CA, Liu H, Lee SS. Altered cellular calcium regulatory systems in a rat model of cirrhotic cardiomyopathy. Gastroenterology. 2001;**121**:1209-1218

[37] Zavecz JH, Bueno O, Maloney RE, ODonnell JM, Roerig SC, Battarbee HD. Cardiac excitation–contraction coupling in the portal hypertensive rat. American Journal of Physiology-Gastrointestinal and Liver Physiology. 2000;**279**:G28-G39

[38] Tavakoli S, Hajrasouliha AR, Jabehdar-Maralani P, Ebrahimi F, Solhpour A, Sadeghipour H, et al. Reduced susceptibility to epinephrine-induced arrhythmias in cirrhotic rats: The roles of nitric oxide and endogenous opioid peptides. Journal of Hepatology. 2007;**46**:432-439

[39] Wong F, Siu S, Liu P, Blendis LM. Brain natriuretic peptide: Is it a predictor of cardiomyopathy in cirrhosis? Clinical Science (London, England). 2001;**101**:621-628

[40] Henriksen JH, Gotze JP, Fuglsang S, Christensen E, Bendtsen F, Møller S. Increased circulating pro-brain natriuretic peptide (proBNP) and brain natriuretic peptide (BNP) in patients with cirrhosis: Relation to cardiovascular dysfunction and severity of disease. Gut. 2003;**52**:1511-1517

[41] Grose RD, Nolan J, Dillon JF, et al. Exercise-induced left ventricular dysfunction in alcoholic and non-alcoholic cirrhosis. Journal of Hepatology. 1995;**22**:326-332

[42] Kelbaek H, Eriksen J, Brynjolf I, et al. Cardiac performance in patients with asymptomatic alcoholic cirrhosis of the liver. The American Journal of Cardiology. 1984;**54**:852-855

[43] Finucci G, Desideri A, Sacerdoti D, et al. Left ventricular diastolic function in liver cirrhosis. Scandinavian Journal of Gastroenterology. 1996;**31**:279-284

[44] Epstein SK, Ciubotaru RL, Zilberberg MD, et al. Analysis of impaired exercise capacity in patients with cirrhosis. Digestive Diseases and Sciences. 1998;**43**:1701-1707

[45] Chayanupatkul M, Liangpunsakul S. Cirrhotic cardiomyopathy: Review of pathophysiology and treatment. Hepatology International. 2014;**8**(3):308-315. DOI: 10.1007/s12072-014-9531-y

[46] Moller S, Henriksen JH. Cardiovascular complications of cirrhosis. Gut. 2008;**57**:268-278

[47] Schenk EA, Cohen J. The heart in chronic alcoholism. Clinical and pathologic findings. Pathologica et Microbiologica (Basel). 1970;**35**:96-104

[48] Nagueh SF, Appleton CP, Gillebert TC, et al. Recommendations for the evaluation of left ventricular diastolic function by echocardiography. European Journal of Echocardiography. 2009;**10**:165-193

[49] Braverman AC, Steiner MA, Picus D, White H. High-output congestive heart failure following transjugular intrahepatic portal-systemic shunting. Chest. 1995;**107**:1467-1469

[50] Huonker M, Schumacher YO, Ochs A, Sorichter S, Keul J, Rossle M. Cardiac function andhaemodynamics in alcoholic cirrhosis and effects of the transjugular intrahepatic portosystemic stent shunt. Gut. 1999;**44**:743-748

[51] Sola E, Gines P. Renal and circulatory dysfunction in cirrhosis: Current management and future perspectives. Journal of Hepatology. 2010;**53**:1135-1145

[52] Schrier RW, Arroyo V, Bernardi M, Epstein M, Henriksen JH, Rodes J. Peripheral arterial vasodilation hypothesis: A proposal for the initiation

of renal sodium and water retention in cirrhosis. Hepatology. 1988;**8**:1151-1157

[53] Kwon HM, Hwang GS. Cardiovascular dysfunction and liver transplantation. Korean Journal of Anesthesiology. 2018;**71**(2):85-91

[54] Kawut SM, Krowka MJ, Trotter JF, et al. Clinical risk factors for portopulmonary hypertension. Hepatology. 2008;**48**:196-203

[55] Ramsay M. Portopulmonary hypertension and hepatopulmonary syndromeand liver transplantation. International Anesthesiology Clinics. 2006;**44**:69-82

[56] Ramsay M. Liver transplantation and pulmonary hypertension: Pathophysiology and management strategies. Current Opinion in Organ Transplantation. 2007;**12**:274-280

[57] Krowka MJ, Plevak DJ, Findlay JY, et al. Pulmonary hemodynamics and perioperative cardiopulmonary-related mortality in patients with portopulmonary hypertension undergoing liver transplantation. Liver Transplantation. 2000;**6**:443-450

[58] Mukhtar NA, Fix OK. Portopulmonary hypertension. Journal of Clinical Gastroenterology. 2011;**45**:703-710

[59] Rodriguez-Roisin R, Krowka M, Herve´ P, Fallon M. Pulmonary-hepatic vascular disorders (PHD). The European Respiratory Journal. 2004;**24**:861-880

[60] Swanson KL, Wiesner RH, Nyberg SL, et al. Survival in portopulmonary hypertension: Mayo clinic experience categorized by treatment subgroups. American Journal of Transplantation. 2008;**8**:2445-2453

[61] Wong F, Liu P, Lilly L, Bomzon A, Blendis L. Role of cardiac structural and functional abnormalities in the pathogenesis of hyperdynamic circulation and renal sodium retention in cirrhosis. Clinical Science (London, England). 1999;**97**:259-267

[62] Nagueh SF, Appleton CP, Gillebert TC, Marino PN, et al. Recommendations for the evaluation of left ventricular diastolic function by echocardiography. Journal of the American Society of Echocardiography. 2009;**22**:107-133

[63] Kasner M, Westermann D, Steendijk P, Gaub R, Wilkenshoff U, et al. Utility of Doppler echocardiography and tissue Doppler imaging in the estimation of diastolic function in heart failure with normal ejection fraction: A comparative Doppler-conductance catheterization study. Circulation. 2007;**116**:637-647

[64] Oki T, Tabata T, Yamada H, Iuchi A. Clinical application of pulsed Doppler tissue imaging for assessing abnormal left ventricular relaxation. The American Journal of Cardiology. 1997;**79**:921-928

[65] Ommen SR, Nishimura RA, Appleton CP, Miller FA, Oh JK, et al. Clinical utility of Doppler echocardiography and tissue Doppler imaging in the estimation of left ventricular filling pressures: A comparative simultaneous Doppler-catheterization study. Circulation. 2000;**102**:1788-1794

[66] Fouad TR, Abdel-Razek WM, Burak KW, Bain VG, Lee SS. Prediction of cardiac complications after liver transplantation. Transplantation. 2009;**87**:763-770

[67] Vitin AA, Tomescu D, Azamfirei L. Hemodynamic optimization strategies in anesthesia care for liver transplantation. In: Liver Cirrhosis–Update and Current Challenges. InTech Co.; 2016, Chapter 9, ISBN: 978-953-51-3310-0. pp. 173-195

[68] Ripoll C, Catalina MV, Yotti R, et al. Cardiac dysfunction during liver transplantation: Incidence and preoperative predictors. Transplantation. 27 Jun 2008;**85**(12):1766-1772. DOI: 10.1097/TP.0b013e318172c936

[69] Feltracco P, Barbieri S, Galligioni H, Michieletto E, Carollo C, Or C. Intensive care management of liver transplanted patients. World Journal of Hepatology. 2011;**3**(3):61-71

[70] Sonny A, Ibrahim A, Schuster A, Jaber WA, Cywinski JB. Impact and persistence of cirrhotic cardiomyopathy after liver transplantation. Clinical Transplantation. 2016;**30**:986-993

[71] Henriksen JH, Bendtsen F, Hansen EF, Møller S. Acute non-selective β-adrenergic blockade reduces prolonged frequency-adjusted QT interval (QTc) in patients with cirrhosis. Journal of Hepatology. 2004;**40**:239-246

[72] Zambruni A, Trevisani F, Caraceni P, Bernardi M. Effect of chronic β-blockade on QT interval in patients with liver cirrhosis. Journal of Hepatology. 2008;**48**:415-421

[73] Pozzi M, Ratti L, Redaelli E, Guidi C, et al. Cardiac, neuroadrenergic, and portal hemodynamic effects of prolonged aldosterone blockade in post-viral child A cirrhosis. The American Journal of Gastroenterology. 2005;**100**:1110-1116

[74] Pitt B. Do diuretics and aldosterone receptor antagonists improve ventricular remodeling? Journal of Cardiac Failure. 2002;**8** (6 Suppl):S491-S493

[75] Reddy K, Mallett S, Peachey T. Venovenous bypass in orthotopic liver transplantation: Time for a rethink? Liver Transplantation. 2005;**11**(7):741-749

[76] Beltran J, Taura P, Grande L, Garcia-Valdecasas JC, Rimola A, Cugat E. Venovenous bypass and liver transplantation. Anesthesia & Analgesia. 1993;**77**:642

[77] Johnson MW, Powelson JA, Auchincloss H Jr, Delmonico FL, Cosimi AB. Selective use of veno-venous bypass in orthotopic liver transplantation. Clinical Transplants. 1996;**10**:181-185

[78] Nadim MK, Annanthapanyasut W, Matsuoka L, Appachu K, Boyajian M, Ji L, et al. Intraoperative hemodialysis during liver transplantation: A decade of experience. Liver Transplantation. 2014;**20**(7):756-764. DOI: 10.1002/lt.23867

[79] Sedra AH, Strum E. The role of intraoperative hemodialysis in liver transplant patients. Current Opinion in Organ Transplantation. 2011;**16**:323-325

[80] Takashi M, Hilmi IA, Planinsic RM, Humar A, Sakai A. Cardiac arrest during adult liver transplantation: A single institution's experience with 1238 deceased donor transplants. Liver Transplantation. 2012;**18**:1430-1439

[81] Fischer W, Bengtsson Y, Scarola S, Cohen E. Methylene blue for vasopressor-resistant vasoplegia syndrome during liver transplantation. Journal of Cardiothoracic and Vascular Anesthesia. 2010;**24**(3):463-466

[82] Mandell MS, Katz JJ, Wachs M, Gill E, Kam I. Circulatory pathophysiology and options in hemodynamic management during adult liver transplantation. Liver Transplantation and Surgery. 1997;**3**:379-387

[83] Vater Y, Levy A, Martay K, Hunter C, Weinbroum AA. Adjuvant drugs for end-stage liver failure and transplantation. Medical Science Monitor. 2004;**10**:RA77-RA88

[84] Ceolotto G, Papparella I, Sticca A, et al. An abnormal gene expression of the -adrenergic system contributes to the pathogenesis of cardiomyopathy in cirrhotic rats. Hepatology. 2008;**48**:1913-1923

Chapter 8

Pharmacotherapy of Hepatic Encephalopathy

Shatha Al-Muhaideb and Aziza A. Ajlan

Abstract

Hepatic encephalopathy (HE) or portosystemic encephalopathy (PSE) is a serious neuropsychiatric disorder resulting from liver failure. It is one of the common complications of liver cirrhosis and portosystemic shunting (PSS). Ammonia accumulation is one of the well-established causes. Ammonia is a by-product of the intestinal bacteria as a result of the breakdown of dietary supplements. In the normal state of the liver, the peripheral hepatocyte contains glutaminase that converts glutamine into glutamate and ammonia; ammonia will be detoxified and converted into urea. The variant manifestations were linked to the severity of HE. A wide range of neurological and psychiatric signs have been reported. The International Society for Hepatic Encephalopathy and Nitrogen Metabolism (ISHEN) uses asterixis (i.e., flapping tremor) as the first clinical sign of HE. Four factors should be taken into consideration to classify and distinguish HE from other conditions: HE type, severity of manifestations following West-Haven Criteria (WHC), HE time course, and presence of precipitating factors. Nonabsorbable disaccharides (lactulose and lactitol) and rifaximin have been the standard of care as first- and second-line therapies, respectively. Non-pharmacological interventions had a crucial role in HE management. Liver transplantation is the ultimate management of hepatic cirrhosis.

Keywords: liver cirrhosis complications, hepatic encephalopathy, hepatic stupor, hepatic coma, portosystemic encephalopathy, hepato-cerebral encephalopathy, hyperammonemia, pharmacotherapy

1. Introduction

Hepatic encephalopathy (HE) or portosystemic encephalopathy (PSE) is a serious neuropsychiatric disorder resulting from liver failure [1]. It is a state of abnormal neurological manifestations ranging from subclinical alterations to coma. It can be classified into three types based on underlying etiology. It is one of the common complications of liver cirrhosis and portosystemic shunting (PSS). HE accounts for 62% mortality rate among cirrhotic patients over 3 years [2]. A description of HE clinical state is as old as the Prognostics and Prosthetics of Hippocrates [3]. The association between jaundice and delirium was linked to cirrhosis as early as the seventeenth century [3]. In the absence of preexisting disease, acute, severe liver failure may cause the brain to swell, with patients becoming comatose and losing brain function altogether. Hepatic encephalopathy in patients with chronic liver disease is revocable and controllable, but new, acute (fulminant) hepatic encephalopathy with speedily mounting blood ammonia values is harder to control due to the diffuse brain edema as well as structural brain-stem injury [4, 5].

Although HE is linked to liver cirrhosis, multifactorial complex pathogenesis is involved but not fully understood.

2. Epidemiology

Over a year, 5 to 7% of cirrhotic patients progress from a compensated state to decompensated stage [4]. The progression of the disease reduces survival by 10 years, with life expectancy around 12 years in patients with compensated liver cirrhosis that drop to 2 years in decompensated end-stage liver disease [4]. Mortality rate among patients in end-stage liver disease was 20% over 1 year. HE is one of the definitions of decompensated liver disease [5]. The incidence of overt HE ranges from 10 to 14% at the time of diagnosis and increases up to 21% at decompensated state and up to 50% in patients post transjugular intrahepatic portosystemic shunt (TIPS). Overall, up to 4% of cirrhotic patients will have HE state sometimes during the disease course. Once the patient develops the first episode of HE, the risk of recurrence increases up to 40% within a year from the first episode [5]. After the first episode of HE, the survival rate at 1 and 3 years was 73% and 38%, respectively [2].

3. Pathophysiology

The exact pathophysiology of HE has not been entirely understood with multiple mechanisms identified as pathological etiologies of HE. Ammonia accumulation is one of the well-described causes [6]. Ammonia is a by-product of the intestinal bacteria as a result of the breakdown of dietary supplements. In the normal state of the liver, the peripheral hepatocyte contains glutaminase that converts glutamine into glutamate and ammonia; ammonia will be detoxified and converted into urea, a product that is easily excreted by the kidneys. In case of liver cirrhosis, ammonia accumulates and is shifted into the systemic circulation leading to the activation of other detoxifying pathways (e.g., skeletal muscle, kidney, and brain). However, overtime ammonia will accumulate [6]. Neurotoxins that prevent the transmission of amino acids and electrolytes across the brain membrane is known [6]. The impact of ammonia on the neurons is directly linked to HE manifestations. This is one of the most targeted mechanisms for HE treatment. At high levels, ammonia will be able to penetrate the blood-brain barrier. Subsequently, glutamine is formed when astrocytic glutamine synthetase converts ammonia and glutamate. This in turn acts as an osmolyte and increases cerebral volume.

Nevertheless, other pathways have been identified including the gamma-aminobutyric acid (GABA), neurosteroids, inflammation, oxidative stress, manganese, zinc deficiency, and intestinal microflora [6]. Further research is needed to understand the magnitude of these factors in HE prognosis and the possibility of targeting those pathways in future therapies.

4. Clinical presentation

The variant manifestations were linked to the severity of HE. A wide range of neurological and psychiatric signs have been reported. The International Society for Hepatic Encephalopathy and Nitrogen Metabolism (ISHEN) uses asterixis (i.e., flapping tremor) as the first clinical sign of HE [7]. The neurological symptoms might be mild to the extent of being undetectable to noticeable behavioral changes progressing to coma. HE may affect psychology, memory, visuospatial ability, and brain electrophysiology [8]. Hence, a series of manifestations are seen including but not limited to apathy, irritability, sleep-wake cycle disturbance, disorientation to time and place, hypertonia, and extrapyramidal dysfunction [9]. It is worth mentioning that none of these manifestations is HE pathognomonic finding.

5. Diagnosis and classification

The wide range of clinical manifestations necessitates a consensus diagnostic and classification criteria. Four factors should be taken into consideration to classify and distinguish HE from other conditions [5]: first, HE type (i.e., Type A resulting from acute liver failure, Type B resulting from PSS, and Type C resulting from liver cirrhosis); second, severity of manifestations where the most commonly used are West-Haven Criteria (WHC) with five grades (**Table 1** Minimal to Grade IV) and ISHEN criteria with two categories (covert and overt HE); third, HE time course: classified into episodic, recurrent (i.e., within 6 months or less), and persistent; and fourth, the presence of precipitating factors (e.g., infections, electrolyte disorder, gastrointestinal bleeding, transjugular intrahepatic portosystemic shunt). In clinical practice settings, WHC is the most useful tool to identify clinical description, but it should be correlated with the case scenario. Multiple neurological and psychometric clinical tests (e.g., portosystemic encephalopathy, critical flicker frequency, and inhibitory control test) have been developed to early identify minimal and covert HE (MHE and CHE), but it needs expert examiner to appropriately interpret results.

Ammonia level alone cannot be used as a sole diagnostic indicator, and it should be assessed within the clinical context. However, if the level is normal, the HE diagnosis is less likely [5]. Computed tomography (CT) scanning of the head could be performed to rule out structural considerations in the differential diagnosis, including intracranial hemorrhage. However, for patients with well-documented liver disease, it might not be necessary.

Grade	Criteria
Grade 0	Lack of detectable changes in personality or behavior, no asterixis
Grade 1	Trivial lack of awareness, euphoria or anxiety, shortened attention span, impaired performance of addition, and asterixis may present
Grade 2	Lethargy or apathy, minimal disorientation for time or place, inappropriate behavior, subtle personality, slurred speech, impaired performance of subtraction
Grade 3	Somnolence to semistupor but responsive to verbal stimuli, confusion, gross disorientation, and asterixis is usually absent
Grade 4	Coma (unresponsive to verbal or noxious stimuli)

Table 1.
West-Haven Criteria (WHC) [2, 5].

6. Management

The principle of HE management involves several steps. Those include airway protection (for patients presenting with coma), treat or prevent precipitating factors, analyze and treat other causes of altered mental status (e.g., hyponatremia, diabetes, thiamin deficiency, intracranial bleeding), and provide pharmacological and non-pharmacological treatments. Different approaches are used to either treat or prevent HE.

6.1 Non-pharmacological treatment and prevention

6.1.1 Protein restrictions

Protein restriction is one of the components of managing patients with HE. As result, cirrhotic patients have higher prevalence of malnutrition [10]. During episodes of overt HE, protein restriction is advised. Once symptoms of HE are resolved, protein intake can be resumed: range 1–1.5 g/kg/day coupled with other therapies. This should be coupled with maintaining energy intakes at 35–40 kcal/kg ideal body weight daily [5].

Protein source may also play a role in management of HE. Vegetable protein with higher fiber content may be preferable to animal protein as it decreases colonic putrefaction [11, 12]. Animal protein contains high amounts of aromatic amino acids; those amino acids can work as substrates to neurotransmitter's tyramine and octopamine, are thought to inhibit dopaminergic neurotransmission, and worsen hepatic encephalopathy [11, 12].

6.1.2 Fecal transplant and probiotics

Fecal microbiota transplant was also reported to have beneficial outcomes reversing the intestinal microbial dysbiosis [13]. Additionally, probiotics have been used as secondary prophylaxis of HE, either as natural probiotics or in a pharmaceutical dosage form [14, 15].

6.1.3 Liver transplantation and artificial support system

Non-pharmacological interventions have a crucial role in HE management. Liver transplantation is the ultimate management of hepatic cirrhosis [5]. However, the complexity and challenges of such approach reduce the feasibility of transplantation. Other interventions may improve overall liver function, e.g., balloon-occluded retrograde transvenous obliteration, taking into consideration the applicability of each procedure on case-by-case manner [16]. Nevertheless, artificial liver support system was reported to have positive impact on overall liver cirrhosis complications, including HE [17, 18].

6.2 Pharmacological treatment and prevention

6.2.1 Non-absorbable disaccharides (lactulose and lactitol)

Lactulose is considered as the first-line therapy and has been in medical use since the 1950s. It is a form of synthesized fructose sugar containing galactose and lactose, while lactitol is a synthetic alcohol sugar consisting of lactose and sorbitol. It has been in the pharmaceutical market since 1987. As non-absorbable nutrients, the normal flora degradation of lactulose or lactitol leads to the reduction in PH toward acidic media in the colon. It will convert ammonia (NH_3) into ammonium (NH_4) that enhances a shift in NH_3 concentration and hence the movement from the blood to the intestine. This will reduce the ammonia level from dietary and endogenous source (**Table 2**). Nevertheless, they act as osmotic

Therapeutic agents*	**Mechanism of action**	**Role in therapy**
Nonabsorbable disaccharides (lactulose and lactitol)	Normal flora degradation of lactulose or lactitol leads to the reduction in PH toward acidic media in the colon. It will convert ammonia (NH_3) into ammonium (NH_4) that enhances a shift in NH_3 concentration and hence the movement from the blood to the intestine	First-line therapy
Rifaximin	Local action of rifaximin inhibits the bacteria protein synthesis via binding to RpoB inhibiting the function of DNA-dependent RNA polymerase	Add-on therapy

**Other therapies do not have a clear role in treatment and can be considered on a case-by-case basis.*

Table 2.
Recommended pharmacological treatment [5].

laxatives that increase water into the intestines and stimulate a bowel movement. Over the years, lactulose and lactitol are used to treat constipation and hyperammonemia. A systematic review assessing the impact of non-absorbable disaccharides on HE outcomes resulted in the inclusion of 22 randomized clinical trials (RCT) evaluating either lactulose or lactitol, neither showing significant difference in clinical outcomes including HE improvement and mortality [19]. Few years later, another systematic review was conducted. They included 38 RCT assessing the effect of either lactulose or lactitol in HE treatment and prevention. There was no significant difference between the two agents, but both of them had a beneficial effect on HE, including serious liver-related adverse events (e.g., variceal bleeding, serious infections, and hepatorenal syndrome), HE recurrence, and overall mortality [20]. The continuation on non-absorbable disaccharides beyond the treatment period had a positive impact on HE recurrence [21, 22]. Generally, both lactulose and lactitol have preferable safety profile and low burden from cost perspectives. However, non-favorable effects such as hypernatremia, hypokalemia, and gastrointestinal side effects have been reported. In lactose-intolerant patients, such side effects might be more pronounced. Polyethylene glycol (PEG) is a promising alternative, but further studies are needed to have robustness positive outcomes of PEG in HE management [23]. For all osmotic laxatives used in HE, two to four bowel motions per day as targeted outcome of therapy used to adjust doses and avoid side effects. Initial dose of 25 mL lactulose given orally every 1–2 hours until the patient has two bowel motions or loose stool can be adjusted accordingly [5]. Continuation on therapy reduces the risk of recurrent HE episode as long as the risk of lactulose overuse is monitored (e.g., dehydration, hypernatremia, severe perianal skin irritation, and even precipitating HE) [5]. No difference between oral and rectal as route of administration, however, based on the clinical context, one of them might be preferable over the other (e.g., comatose patient) [24].

6.2.2 Antibiotics

Antibiotics' role in HE management fills within the inhibition of ammonia-producing colonic bacteria. Rifaximin is a poorly absorbed bactericidal antibiotic (rifamycins). It is available in the market since 2004, and the Food and Drug Administration (FDA) approval for patients with liver disease was obtained in 2010. Rifaximin has a wide-spectrum antibacterial activity including anaerobic species. Local action of rifaximin inhibits the bacteria protein synthesis via binding to RpoB inhibiting the function of DNA-dependent RNA polymerase. At dose of 550 mg PO twice daily, it was effective in HE treatment and prevention of recurrent episode. However, it was used as add-on therapy where majority of participants were using lactulose [25, 26] (**Table 2**). Different antibiotics have been used in HE management including neomycin, metronidazole, and vancomycin [27]. Neomycin is an aminoglycoside with controversy outcomes regarding its efficacy in HE. Antibacterial activity and glutaminase inhibition are the proposed mechanisms of neomycin effect in HE [27]. In attempt to find safer, effective, and more tolerable alternative, both metronidazole and vancomycin have been studied. Oral metronidazole is used with success, yet peripheral neuropathy may occur with long-term therapy. Limited studies were conducted in patients with poor response to lactulose monotherapy and showed improved response [27]. Although the FDA approved it, taking into consideration the safety profile of those agents (e.g., ototoxicity and neurotoxicity) and the risk of resistance development favors rifaximin over other antibiotics, although peripheral edema, central nervous system (CNS) side effects, and gastrointestinal intolerance have been reported with rifaximin. Published data on rifaximin cost-effectiveness showed that rifaximin alone was not cost-effective. Hence, it is not recommended as first-line therapy. However, in patients who are not responding to lactulose/lactitol, the addition of rifaximin may reduce hospitalization and prevent recurrence [28–30]. The availability of a generic rifaximin may change the cost-effectiveness outcomes.

6.2.3 L-ornithine-L-aspartate (LOLA)

The efficacy of intravenous L-ornithine L-aspartate (LOLA) as monotherapy in MHE was assessed in a RCT; it showed improved ammonia level and mental states [31]. In a meta-analysis of eight randomized trials with 646 patients in total, LOLA had a significant effect on improvement of hepatic encephalopathy total (RR, 1.49; 95% confidence interval [CI], 1.10 to 2.01) and overt HE (RR, 1.33; 95% CI, 1.04 to 1.69) [32]. LOLA has not been compared directly to active treatment (e.g., lactulose).

6.2.4 Glycerol phenylbutyrate (GPB)

Metabolic ammonia scavengers (e.g., benzoate, phenyl acetate, and glyceryl phenylbutyrate) have been used in genetic disorders involving urea cycle. Such disorders result in hyperammonemia, and such therapeutic agents may exert a possible treatment option [33]. In a randomized, double-blind, placebo-controlled phase II trial enrolling 178 patients with cirrhosis (including patients who were on lactulose ± rifaximin), GPB, dosed at 6 mL orally twice daily, significantly reduced the proportion of patients who experienced an HE event (21% versus 36%; $P = 0.02$), time to first event (hazard ratio [HR] = 0.56; $P < 0.05$), as well as total events (35 versus 57; $P = 0.04$) and was associated with fewer HE hospitalizations (13 versus 25; $P = 0.06$) [33]. Further trails are still required to validate the results. Moreover, the current cost of the drug may still be a barrier to its use at a larger scale.

6.2.5 Branched-chain amino acids (BCAA)

Branched-chain amino acids (BCAA) classified into proteinogenic (i.e., leucine, isoleucine, and valine) and non-proteinogenic (i.e., 2-aminoisobutyric acid) are essential amino acids. In limited clinical trials, BCAA had a beneficial impact on HE outcomes in addition to standard therapy. However, this positive effect was limited to oral dosage forms but not the intravenous formulation. BCAA had no impact on mortality, quality of life, or nutritional parameters; additional trials to evaluate such outcomes are needed [34–36].

6.2.6 Zinc supplementation

Zinc deficiency is common in cirrhotic patients. In case of documented deficiency, oral zinc supplementation can improve performance, but it did not affect the risk of recurrence [37]. Hyperammonemia could improve with zinc administration as it increases the activity of ornithine transcarbamylase, an enzyme in the urea cycle. Afterward, the increase in ureagenesis leads to the loss of ammonia ions. Further studies are needed to understand the possible role of micronutrient supplementation on long-term HE outcomes.

6.2.7 Flumazenil

Flumazenil is an antidote to reverse benzodiazepine toxicity by competitively binding to the benzodiazepine receptor site. Symptoms of benzodiazepine toxicity may overlap with HE (e.g., confusion, anxiety, and unresponsiveness). Flumazenil can be used as a diagnostic aid to differentiate between the two conditions [5].

6.2.8 Other therapies

Other therapies have not been assessed extensively in HE management (e.g., albumin and glutaminase inhibitors). Such alternatives had promising outcomes encouraging further research in this area. Albumin intravenous administration did not impact HE directly but improved survival post-discharge [38]. Glutaminase inhibition is a promising target of drug therapy in HE management. It could be a new era of research that may change HE management principle but nothing solid yet [39].

L-Carnitine was found to improve HE symptoms in several small studies of patients with cirrhosis. The exact mechanism remains unclear. One of the proposed mechanisms is that it may work by improving blood ammonia levels or centrally perhaps by decreasing brain ammonia uptake [40].

Dopamine agonists (e.g., levodopa or bromocriptine) are shown to result in improvement in clinical and electroencephalographic findings in anecdotal reports and small studies. If these results are confirmed at larger studies, it may lead to clinical recommendations.

7. Conclusion

HE is a reversible clinical syndrome with a wide range of manifestations, which will negatively impact patient quality of life if mismanaged. Different management approaches have been developed. The most appropriate treatment should be applied on case-by-case fashion.

Conflict of interest

The author declares no conflict of interest.

Author details

Shatha Al-Muhaideb and Aziza A. Ajlan*
King Faisal Specialist Hospital and Research Centre, Riyadh, Saudi Arabia

*Address all correspondence to: aajlan@kfshrc.edu.sa

References

[1] Butterworth R. Neurosteroids in hepatic encephalopathy: Novel insights and new therapeutic opportunities. The Journal of Steroid Biochemistry and Molecular Biology. 2016;**160**:94-97

[2] Bustamante J, Rimola A, Ventura P, et al. Prognostic significance of hepatic encephalopathy in patients with cirrhosis. Journal of Hepatology. 1999;**30**(5):890-895

[3] Amodio P. Hepatic encephalopathy: Historical remarks. Journal of Clinical and Experimental Hepatology. 2015;**5**(1):4-6

[4] D'Amico G, Garcia-Tsao G, Pagliaro L. Natural history and prognostic indicators of survival in cirrhosis: A systematic review of 118 studies. Journal of Hepatology. 2006;**44**:217-231

[5] Vilstrup H, Amodio P, Bajaj J, et al. Hepatic encephalopathy in chronic liver disease: 2014 practice guideline by the American Association for the Study of Liver Diseases and the European Association for the Study of the Liver. Hepatology. 2014;**60**(2):715-735

[6] Savlan I, Liakina V, Valantinas J. Concise review of current concepts on nomenclature and pathophysiology of hepatic encephalopathy. Medicina. 2014;**50**:75-81

[7] Bajaj J, Wade J, Sanyal A. Spectrum of neurocognitive impairment in cirrhosis: Implications for the assessment of hepatic encephalopathy. Hepatology. 2009;**50**(6):2014-2021

[8] Amodio P, Montagnese S, Gatta A, et al. Characteristics of minimal hepatic encephalopathy. Metabolic Brain Disease. 2004;**19**(3):253-267

[9] Adams R, Foley J. The neurological disorder associated with liver disease. Research Publications - Association for Research in Nervous and Mental Disease. 1953;**32**:198-237

[10] Amodio P, Bemeur C, Butterworth R, et al. The nutritional management of hepatic encephalopathy in patients with cirrhosis: International Society for Hepatic Encephalopathy and Nitrogen Metabolism Consensus. Hepatology. 2013;**58**:325-336

[11] Plauth M, Merli M, Kondrup J, et al. ESPEN guidelines for nutrition in liver disease and transplantation. Clinical Nutrition. 1997;**16**:43-55

[12] Dallas DC, Sanctuary MR, Qu Y, et al. Personalizing protein nourishment. Critical Reviews in Food Science and Nutrition. 2017;**57**(15):3313-3331

[13] Mehta R, Kabrawala M, Nandwani S, et al. Preliminary experience with single fecal microbiota transplant for treatment of recurrent overt hepatic encephalopathy–A case series. Indian Journal of Gastroenterology. 2018;**37**(6):559-562. Accessed on https://rd.springer.com/article/10.1007%2Fs12664-018-0906-1. Accessed 16th Dec. 2018

[14] Vera C, Illanes A. Lactose-derived nondigestible oligosaccharides and other high added-value products. 2016. DOI: 10.1016/B978-0-12-802724-0.00003-2

[15] Agrawal A, Sharma BC, Sharma P, et al. Trial of lactulose, probiotics, and no therapy. The American Journal of Gastroenterology. 2012;**107**(7):1043-1050

[16] Nakazawa M, Imai Y, Uchiya H, et al. Balloon-occluded retrograde transvenous obliteration as a procedure to improve liver function in patients with decompensated cirrhosis. JGH Open. 2017:127-133

[17] Wang Y, Zhu X, Feng D, Wu B. Artificial liver support system for acute-on-chronic liver failure combined with successful liver transplantation in stage III-IV hepatic encephalopathy: An analysis of 14 cases. Zhonghua Gan Zang Bing Za Zhi. 2018;**26**(9):676-679

[18] Mac Donald A, Karvellas C. Emerging role of extracorporeal support in acute and acute-on-chronic liver failure: Recent developments. Seminars in Respiratory and Critical Care Medicine. 2018;**39**(5):625-634

[19] Als-Nielsen B, Gluud LL, Gluud C. Non-absorbable disaccharides for hepatic encephalopathy: Systematic review of randomized trials. BMJ. 2004:1-6

[20] Gluud L, Vilstrup H, Morgan M. Nonabsorbable disaccharides for hepatic encephalopathy: A systematic review and meta-analysis. Hepatology. 2016;**64**(3):908-922

[21] Bajaj J, Gillevet P, Patel N, et al. A longitudinal systems biology analysis of lactulose withdrawal in hepatic encephalopathy. Metabolic Brain Disease. 2012;**27**(2):2015-2215

[22] Bajaj J, Sanyal A, Bell D, et al. Predictors of the recurrence of hepatic encephalopathy in lactulose-treated patients. Alimentary Pharmacology & Therapeutics. 2010;**31**(9):1012-1017

[23] Rahimi R, Singal A, Cuthbert J, Rockey D. Lactulose vs polyethylene glycol 3350 – Electrolyte solution for treatment of overt hepatic encephalopathy: The HELP randomized clinical trial. JAMA Internal Medicine. 2014;**174**(11):1727-1733

[24] Al Sibae MR, McGuire BM. Current trends in the treatment of hepatic encephalopathy. Therapeutics and Clinical Risk Management. 2009;**5**:617-626

[25] Bass NM, Mullen KD, Sanyal A, et al. Rifaximin treatment in hepatic encephalopathy. NEJM. 2010;**362**(12):1071-1081

[26] Koo H, DuPont H. Rifaximin: A unique gastrointestinal-selective antibiotic for enteric diseases. Current Opinion in Gastroenterology. 2010;**26**(1):17-25

[27] Patidar K, Bajaj J. Antibiotics for the treatment of hepatic encephalopathy. Metabolic Brain Disease. 2013;**28**(2):307-312

[28] Neff G, Zachry W. Systematic review of the economic burden of overt hepatic encephalopathy and pharmacoeconomic impact of rifaximin. PharmacoEconomics. 2018;**36**:809-822

[29] Huang E, Esrailian E, Spiegel B. The cost-effectiveness and budget impact of competing therapies in hepatic encephalopathy-a decision analysis. Alimentary Pharmacology & Therapeutics. 2007;**26**(8):1147-1161

[30] Agrawal A, Sharma BC, Sharma P, et al. Secondary prophylaxis of hepatic encephalopathy in cirrhosis: An open-label, randomized controlled trial of lactulose, probiotics, and no therapy. American Journal of Gastroenterology. 2012;**107**(7):1043-1050. DOI: 10.1038/ajg.2012.113

[31] Kircheis G, Nilius R, Held C, et al. Therapeutic efficacy of L-ornithine-L-aspartate infusions in patients with cirrhosis and hepatic encephalopathy: Results of a placebo-controlled, double-blind study. Hepatology. 1997;**25**(6):1351-1360

[32] Bai M, Yang Z, Qi X, et al. L-ornithine-l-aspartate for hepatic encephalopathy in patients with cirrhosis: A meta-analysis of randomized controlled trials. Journal of Gastroenterology and Hepatology.

2013;**28**(5):783-792. DOI: 10.1111/jgh.12142

[33] Rockey D, Vierling J, Mantry P, et al. Randomized, double-blind, controlled study of glycerol phenylbutyrate in hepatic encephalopathy. Hepatology. 2014;**59**(3):1073-1083

[34] Gluud LL, Dam G, Borre M, et al. Lactulose, rifaximin, or branched chain amino acids for hepatic encephalopathy: What is the evidence? Metabolic Brain Disease. 2013;**28**(2):221-225

[35] Gluud LL, Dam G, Borre M, et al. Oral branched-chain amino acids have a beneficial effect on manifestations of hepatic encephalopathy in a systemic review with meta-analyses of randomized controlled trials. The Journal of Nutrition. 2013;**143**(8):1263-1268

[36] Naylor C, O'Rourke K, Detsky A, Baker J. Parenteral nutrition with branched-chain amino acids in hepatic encephalopathy: A meta-analysis. Gastroenterology. 1989;**97**(4):1033-1042

[37] Chavez-Tapia NC, Cesar-Arce A, Barrientos-Gutiérrez T, et al. A systematic review and meta-analysis of the use of oral zinc in the treatment of hepatic encephalopathy. Nutrition Journal. 2013;**12**(74):1-6

[38] Simón-Talero M, García-Martínez R, Torrens M, et al. Effects of intravenous albumin in patients with cirrhosis and episodic hepatic encephalopathy: A randomized double-blind study. Journal of Hepatology. 2013;**59**(6):1184-1192

[39] Díaz-Herrero MM, del Campo JA, Carbonero-Aguilar P, et al. THDP17 decreases ammonia production through glutaminase inhibition: A new drug for hepatic encephalopathy therapy. PLoS One. 2014;**9**(10):1-8

[40] Malaguarnera M. Acetyl-L-carnitine in hepatic encephalopathy. Metabolic Brain Disease. 2013;**28**(2):193-199

Section 3

Cirrhosis and Liver Transplantation: New Perspectives

Chapter 9

New Perspectives on the Use of Sub-Optimal Donor Livers

Maria Eugenia Cornide-Petronio, Mariana Mendes-Braz, Mónica B. Jiménez-Castro, Jordi Gracia-Sancho and Carmen Peralta

Abstract

Liver transplantation is the therapy of choice for patients with end-stage liver disease. However, a shortage of donor organs remains a major obstacle to the widespread application of liver transplantation. To overcome this problem, transplant centers have developed strategies to expand the organ donor pool, including the routine use of sub-optimal donor livers. However, these have an increased risk of initial poor function or primary non-function that may cause greater risk of morbidity in the recipient. This chapter aims to describe the pathophysiological changes that may occur in sub-optimal donor livers, focusing on viral infections, since, after transplantation, infection of the graft is almost universal and can lead to chronic hepatitis, cirrhosis, and graft failure. The different experimental models as well as the clinical outcomes of the transplantation of sub-optimal donor livers with viral infections will be discussed. Such information may be useful to guide the design of better experimental models than those described to date as well as the effective use of sub-optimal livers with successful clinical application.

Keywords: liver transplantation, fibrosis, HCV, HBC, treatment

1. Introduction

End-stage liver disease is associated with high morbidity and mortality, and the only cure is orthotopic liver transplantation (LT). The number of people awaiting LT continues to increase [1] and exceeds the number of available grafts. Between 20 and 30% of patients waiting for LT will die on the waiting list or are delisted because of disease progression [2]. The large imbalance between the growing pool of potential LT recipients and the scarcity of donor organs has led to efforts to maximize the number of existing donors and identify possible new donors based on the use of liver grafts that are currently considered unsuitable for transplant due to their pathological condition [3]. To expand the potential donor pool, the clinical and scientific community is continually modifying the criteria for an acceptable liver donor and is turning to marginal or extended-criteria donors to meet waiting list demands [4]. Thus organs infected with hepatitis B (HBV) or C virus (HCV) are increasingly being used [5], although the risk to recipients of using such grafts remains unclear [6].

Over 2 billion people across the world have serological evidence of present or past infection with HBV and more than 350 million individuals are estimated to be chronically infected [7]. It is estimated that 2–15% of liver donors are anti-hepatitis B core antigen (anti-HBc) positive. The proportion of positive anti-HBc livers in donors aged 60 years or over may rise to as much as 25% [8, 9]. Acquisition of HBV remains a concern after LT because the majority of infections occur via transmission by the donor liver [10], but some donors with past exposure to HBV infection can be used selectively in some recipients [3].

HCV is the most common indication for LT, and at current it accounts for 40–50% of individuals on waiting lists [11–13]. About 5% of all potential organ donors are positive for HCV [14]. To date, one of the most controversial issues regarding extended-criteria donors has revolved around the potential positive impact of HCV-infected donors on short-term outcomes [15]. In Europe, the prevalence of anti-HBc-positive grafts reaches as much as 10% in some regions [5, 9, 16]. A multivariate analysis of the United Network for Organ Sharing database revealed that the use of anti-HBc-positive grafts is not an independent determinant of graft or patient survival [17]. There is a trend towards increasing the use of HCV-positive donors [18]. One-year patient survival rates of 97% have been reported in recipients of HCV-infected livers compared with rates of 87% for recipients of organs meeting the United Network for Organ Sharing-approved criteria, with no differences in surgical conditions including warm and cold ischemia times between the two groups [19].

A significant number of organ donors have viral infections and the effect of using such organs is an important and timely question. In this chapter we describe the pathophysiological changes in sub-optimal donor livers with viral infections. In addition, post-operative outcomes after LT using sub-optimal donor livers with viral infections will be discussed. Therefore, I/R injury, hepatic inflammation and the different treatments used in recipients of donor livers with viral infections will be reviewed. Finally, we give details of the different experimental models of LT with viral infections. All of this may be useful to guide the design of appropriate experimental models of LT that resemble clinical conditions as much as possible, together with addressing the effective use of sub-optimal livers for transplant and the development of new protective strategies in the clinical setting of LT.

2. Sub-optimal donor and fibrosis progression

Many studies have reported the transmission of HBV from liver allografts of hepatitis B surface antigen (HBsAg)-negative, anti-HBc-positive donors [10, 20–28]. HBV within hepatocytes and passenger leukocytes in the anti-HBc allograft can be the source of infection in the HBsAg recipient [29]. It has been shown that employing liver grafts from these donors can transmit HBV infections to HBsAg-negative recipients and result in de novo hepatitis B at rates that are estimated to vary from 33 to 78% after LT in the absence of antiviral prophylaxis [8, 10, 21]. Similarly, there are many reports of the presence of occult HBV infection in HBsAg/anti-HBc donors. Meanwhile, detectable quantities of HBV DNA have been found to be present in only 5–10% of anti-HBc immunocompetent patients, irrespective of their anti-HBs status [30]. The replication capacity of HBV in the anti-HBc liver allograft is significantly increased after LT when recipients are administered high-dose steroids [29]. Several molecular mechanisms have been proposed to explain increased HBV replication in these patients: (1) a glucocorticoid-responsive element in the HBV genome and stimulation of HBV-dependent transcription by glucocorticoids [31]; (2) immunosuppression after LT suppresses virus-specific immune responses whereby after LT wild-type HBV is more frequently re-selected and this can result in better replication fitness of the virus; (3) mutations selected in the HBV preS region result in a cytotoxic HBV strain, which is associated with cholestatic hepatitis [32–34]. HBV infection leads to graft damage in most cases [8]. It has been speculated that a liver that already hosts occult HBV infection, as is the case in the majority of HBcAb-positive donors [35], is particularly liable to suffer rapidly progressive damage when infected by HCV when it encounters immunosuppression for LT [36]. Some studies found that the survival of recipients of anti-HBc livers was significantly reduced 4 years after LT compared with recipients of anti-HBc-negative livers [8, 10]. With a post-LT follow-up of 2–4 years, a minority of transplant recipients developed fibrosing cholestatic hepatitis or cirrhosis leading to allograft failure [37].

Recurrence rates of hepatitis C, manifested by mild chronic hepatitis, fibrosis or cirrhosis, have been reported to be 54.55% in HCV-positive donor grafts when compared with 41.74% in HCV-negative grafts [38]. Marroquin [39] showed that patient survival at 2 years was significantly higher in HCV-positive recipients of HCV-positive grafts than in HCV-positive recipients of HCV-negative grafts (90 vs. 70%). In contrast, other studies indicated that in patients with HCV-related liver disease, there was no significant difference in survival between patients who received an HCV-negative graft and those who received an HCV-negative graft [40]. Khapra et al. [41] suggested that patients receiving HCV-positive donor organs develop more fibrosis over time than those receiving HCV-negative grafts. Wang et al. [42] reported that recipients show progression in liver inflammation grade or fibrosis stage regardless of the HCV status of the donors, although a higher stage of liver inflammation and fibrosis was found in HCV-positive graft recipients at follow-up. Although histological injury in the allograft owing to HCV is exceedingly common, progression of HCV is variable: some individuals experience indolent disease, whereas others progress rapidly to cirrhosis and liver failure [43]. Recently, donor age has been recognized to play an important role after LT with HCV-positive grafts. Khapra et al. [41] reported that HCV-positive grafts aged ≥50 years showed higher rates of graft failure and death among HCV-positive recipients compared to HCV-negative grafts from donors of the same ages. In addition, HCV-positive grafts from advanced-age donors showed more advanced fibrosis than those from younger donors [44].

3. I/R injury and organ dysfunction

Ischemia-reperfusion (I/R) injury, a phenomenon in which cellular damage in a hypoxic organ is accentuated following the restoration of oxygen delivery [45–47], is a multifactorial process associated with organ dysfunction of liver failure after LT. Early graft dysfunction affects up to 22% of liver allografts, with up to 6% of patients developing primary graft non-function and requiring retransplantation [48]. The association of I/R injury with the severity of HCV has been reported by several authors but with conflicting results, since I/R may or may not influence virus recurrence [49]. Although I/R injury is the underlying cause of graft dysfunction in marginal organs [4], it remains an unexplored issue in HBV and HCV grafts from donors.

The process of organ harvesting, cold storage and reperfusion is itself damaging, causing significant oxidative injury that can result in primary nonfunction or increase immunogenicity, prejudicing long-term graft survival [50, 51]. The duration of ischemic rewarming during implantation surgery is a risk factor for the severity of recurrent HCV disease after LT. In patients with hepatitis submitted to LT, the calculated risk for recurrent HCV disease post-LT is 19% if the ischemic time is 30 min versus 65% if this time extends to 90 min [52]. Rewarming ischemic injury appears to cause severe injury that enhances reinfection of the allograft with HCV after reperfusion, eventually leading to hepatic fibrosis and cirrhosis in some patients. Conversely, it has also been reported that cold ischemia time was not a significant risk factor for recurrent HCV infection after LT [53]. Indeed, the authors indicated that rewarming duration during implantation of <10 min was associated with minimal recurrence, whereas a duration of >70 min was associated with moderate to severe recurrent hepatitis. This finding was supported by Velidedeoglu et al. [54] in a United Network for Organ Sharing database study that showed that a warm ischemia time of >90 min was associated with decreased graft survival in HCV-positive individuals [53].

The ischemia-reperfusion procedure itself causes apoptosis, so-called programmed cell death, in the first stages after LT [55], and it can be exacerbated by immunosuppressive drugs used in LT [56]. Balliardini et al. [56] mentioned that both hepatocellular apoptosis and cell proliferation are correlated with HCV infection. Sung et al. [57] suggested that HCV may also stimulate cell growth to counter the apoptosis and thus complete the replication cycle of HCV and produce infectious viral particles. Because the primary target cell for HCV replication in vivo is thought to be the hepatocyte, events that lead to hepatocyte proliferation may enhance HCV replication. Alternatively, HCV core proteins have been shown to interact with cellular promoters and regulators of cell growth, which may affect liver regeneration [58]. All these data suggest that liver regeneration associated with the processes associated with living related LT might affect HCV recurrence. Similarly, I/R injury associated with LT from brain dead donors is associated with apoptosis, whereas HCV is able to counteract apoptosis to increase hepatocyte proliferation. Further studies will be required to elucidate the effect of I/R on HCV recurrence as well as the effects of HCV on hepatic I/R injury associated with LT.

4. Hepatic donor inflammation in response to viral infection

The relationship between hepatocellular injury, hepatic regeneration, viral replicative activity, HCV antigen expression, and the pathologic host response remains unproven. Increased allograft damage is related to enhanced levels of known immune modulators, including interleukines 6 and 10. These cytokines are released in the milieu of injured or proliferating cells and it is known that they participate in the pathogenesis of HCV via increased viral activity, exaggerated host response, or both [59, 60]. Recurrent HCV is characterized by hepatocellular damage, infiltration of inflammatory cells into the liver, and tissue remodeling that ultimately results in progressive fibrosis and cirrhosis. Infiltrating inflammatory cells at the sites of liver injury secrete chemokines that stimulate hepatic stellate cells, these in turn proliferate and produce extracellular matrix proteins. These stellate cells are key players in recurrent HCV and can be activated by a number of stimuli in the liver transplant setting: production of ROS, secretion of cytokines by immune cells (acute rejection, CMV infection), hyperglycemia, and chronic cholestasis (biliary complications). The combination of a variety of factors explains the accelerated progression of fibrosis in HCV-infected liver transplant recipients [61]. Meanwhile, it should also be considered that the factors mentioned above are all generated as a consequence of hepatic I/R. Thus, it can be hypothesized that the mechanisms involved in hepatic I/R may exacerbate the negative post-operative outcomes induced by virus infection.

The mechanism by which the identified factors exert their undesirable effect on HCV recurrence presumably involves host-viral interactions. Since HCV is not directly cytopathic, HCV damage must be mediated by the host immune response. Both CD4- and CD8-positive T-cells participate in the recognition of HCV peptide displayed by infected hepatocytes [62]. In studies using an animal model of acute hepadnavirus infection, using woodchuck HBV, Guo et al. [63] found that viral clearance occurred following the appearance of CD4 and CD8 T-cells as well as the production of interferon gamma and tumor necrosis factor alpha within the infected liver. This was accompanied by a significant increase in apoptosis and regeneration of hepatocytes. HCV infection initiates a specific host response that is ineffective at clearing virus and results in hepatic cellular damage in a nonspecific fashion [53, 64]. The recurrence of HCV is accelerated after LT as a result of high viral loads and an exaggeration of this host response, which occurs even in the presence of exogenous immunosuppression. The alloimmune response and I/R injury may also contribute [53, 65]. Despite the limited information on inflammation and post-transplant viral recurrence, there is a need for a greater understanding of the relationship between the virus and inflammatory processes associated with either I/R or virus infection by itself. This can progress to irreversible liver damage, and is also a relevant issue for the livers of donors infected by virus (HBV and HCV), which are usually in a constant inflammatory state.

5. Viral kinetics and target treatment

Despite being widely described in the literature, viral kinetics before, during and after LT using donor grafts with viral hepatitis has never been analyzed. The subject has only been considered in healthy livers transplanted into recipients with hepatitis. Thus investigations have mainly focused on the life cycle of the viruses and the recurrence of hepatitis.

Donor	Therapy in recipients		Effect
	Before LT	After LT	
Anti-HBc(+) donors [76]	Vaccination with recombinant hepatitis B	Lamivudine	Prevention of de novo HBV infection.
Anti-HBc(+) donors [77]	None	HBV immune globulin plus Lamivudine	Infection successfully managed Survival 100%
Anti-HBc(+) donors [29]	HBV immune globulin	Lamivudine	Prevention of recurrent or de novo infection
Anti-HBc(+) donors [78]	None	HBV immune globulin plus Lamivudine	Prevention of HBV transmission
Anti-HBc(+) donors [79]	Lamivudine or lamivudine plus adefovir	Lamivudine	Prevention of infection development.
Anti-HBc(+) donors [80]	HBV immune globulin	HBV immune globulin plus Lamivudine	Prevention of recurrent infection
Anti-HBc(+) donors [81]	HBV immune globulin	HBV immune globulin vaccination (recombinant)	Minimize the possibility of HBV recurrence
Anti-HBc(+) donors [82]	HBV immune globulin	HBV immune globulin plus Lamivudine	De novo HBV reactivation during HBV immune globulin prophylaxis Lamivudine resulted in virus clearance
Anti-HBc(+) donors [83]	HBV immune globulin	HBV immune globulin plus Lamivudine	Prevention of HBV recurrence

Donor	Therapy in recipients		Effect
	Before LT	**After LT**	
Anti-HBc(+) donors [84]	HBV immune globulin	HBV immune globulin	HBsAg levels became positive
		HBV immune globulin plus Lamivudine	HBsAg-positive
		HBV immune globulin plus lamivudine plus famciclovir	HBsAg-positive
		Lamivudine plus interferon alpha	Serum HBV DNA decreased, but remained positive
		Lamivudine plus adefovir	Hepatitis B e antigen status converted to seronegative
HCV-positive [85]	None	DAA therapy	Increases in life expectancy
HCV-positive [86]	None	DAA therapy	Prevention of HBV recurrence
HCV-positive [87]	None	Ledipasvir and sofosbuvir	Prevention of HCV recurrence

LT, liver transplantation; DAA, direct-acting antivirals; HBV, hepatitis B virus; HCV, hepatitis C virus; HBc, hepatitis B core antigen (anti-HBc); HBsAg, hepatitis B surface antigen.

Table 1.
Pharmacological strategies used in patient after or before the transplantation.

In patients with hepatitis undergoing LT, HCV viral load decreases during the anhepatic phase and after graft reperfusion because of a lack of virus production, blood loss, and hepatic viral clearance. Despite the decline in viral load, hepatitis C virions continue to circulate and rapidly infect the new graft. HCV replication in the liver graft begins within a few hours after LT in most patients [66], and viral load increases as early as 12 h after graft reperfusion. The rapid increase in HCV viral load indicates that viral replication is highly efficient after LT and proves the high capacity of HCV to adapt to a completely new environment. However, HCV kinetics did not follow the same pattern in all patients. Differences in the immunosuppressive regimen appeared to influence HCV kinetics immediately after LT [66]. In fact, HCV-RNA concentrations increased rapidly in patients receiving corticosteroids as part of their immunosuppressive therapy [67–69], whereas they continued to decrease in most patients who were not receiving corticosteroids. Although this observation requires confirmation in further studies, it is possible that some immunosuppressive regimens might be more appropriate in the case of early antiviral therapy to eradicate HCV [66]. Powers et al. [70] estimated that viral resurgence begins when much less than 1% of the engrafted liver's hepatocytes are infected, suggesting that antiviral therapy should begin soon after, or before, LT in order to prevent or delay reinfection.

Table 1 summarizes the pharmacological strategies used in patients before and after LT.

6. Experimental models

To the best of our knowledge, most of the current experimental models of hepatitis do not focus on LT. The only two experimental studies involving hepatitis and LT were by Dahmen et al. [71, 72], and both report severe hepatitis virus reinfection after woodchuck LT (**Table 2**). However, both studies focused on vaccines and not on the effects of I/R on viral infections after LT.

Cold ischemia	Anhepatic	Donor	Receptor	Alterations after LT
<5 h	<40 min	WHV negative	WHV positive	Vascular rejection Severe vacuolar and fatty degeneration Lymphocytic infiltrates and vacuolar degeneration in bile duct
Data not shown	Data not shown	WHV negative + vaccine	WHV positive	Cholangitis was less severe Moderate but stable jaundice Low amounts of viral particles

WHV, woodchuck hepatitis virus.

Table 2.
Experimental studies with hepatitis virus reinfection after liver transplantation.

7. Conclusion

A shortage of donor organs remains a major obstacle to the widespread application of LT in patients with end-stage liver disease [73, 74]. This shortage could be alleviated by routine use of sub-optimal donor livers including those from donors with viral infections, although infection of the graft is almost universal and can lead to chronic hepatitis, cirrhosis, and graft failure. As stated in this chapter, studies on LT using sub-optimal donor grafts with viral infections have mainly focused on survival and the recurrence rates of hepatitis. In addition, although I/R injury is the underlying cause of graft dysfunction in sub-optimal donor livers with viral infections [4], it remains an unexplored issue in recipients transplanted with HBV and HCV grafts. It should be considered that the mechanisms involved in hepatic I/R depend on the conditions used during surgery, such as the period of ischemia (ranging from minutes to days) and the subclinical condition of the graft (healthy, sub-optimal, aged, etc.). However, clinical studies that focus on the pathological effects of I/R were only performed in recipients with viral infections from healthy liver grafts. In our view, multicenter clinical studies and experimental studies of LT using grafts with viral infections are needed to identify the inflammation associated with I/R and that induced by virus infection. The clinical application of strategies designed to increase the use of sub-optimal liver grafts with virus infection will depend on the use of experimental models of LT using donors with viral infections that resemble clinical conditions as much as possible [75]. We recognize that this may be difficult; however, multidisciplinary research groups should devote additional efforts to better understand the pathophysiology of LT using donors with viral infections to ultimately develop effective therapeutic strategies aimed at improving graft viability and at significantly increasing the organ donor pool.

Acknowledgements

This research was supported by the Ministerio de Economía y Competitividad (project grant SAF-2015-64857-R) Madrid, Spain; the European Union (FondosFeder, "una manera de hacer Europa"); by CERCA Program/Generalitat de Catalunya; by the Secretaria d'Universitats i Recerca (Grant 2017SGR-551) Barcelona, Spain. ME Cornide-Petronio has a Sara Borrell contract from the Instituto de Salud Carlos III (Grant CD15/00129), Madrid, Spain. M Mendes-Braz is the recipient of a fellowship from São Paulo Research Foundation (Grant 2018/04625-9), São Paulo, Brazil. MB Jiménez-Castro has a contract from the Programa de Promoción del talento y su empleabilidad from the Ministerio de Economía y Competitividad

(Grant EMP-TU-2015-4167), Madrid, Spain. J Gracia-Sancho received continuous funding from the Instituto de Salud Carlos III (currently FIS PI17/00012) & the CIBEREHD, from Ministerio de Ciencia, Innovación y Universidades.

Conflict of interest

The authors declare that they have no conflict of interest.

Author details

Maria Eugenia Cornide-Petronio[1], Mariana Mendes-Braz[1,2], Mónica B. Jiménez-Castro[3], Jordi Gracia-Sancho[4] and Carmen Peralta[1,5,6*]

1 Institut d'Investigacions Biomèdiques August Pi i Sunyer (IDIBAPS), Barcelona, Spain

2 Laboratory of Immunoendocrinology, Department of Clinical and Toxicological Analyses, School of Pharmaceutical Sciences of University Sao Paulo (FCF/USP), São Paulo, SP, Brazil

3 Transplant Biomedicals, S.L., Barcelona, Spain

4 Barcelona Hepatic Hemodynamic Laboratory, Institut d'Investigacions Biomèdiques August Pi i Sunyer (IDIBAPS), Hospital Clínic de Barcelona, Centro de Investigaciones Biomédicas en Red en Enfermedades Hepáticas y Digestivas (CIBEREHD), Barcelona, Spain

5 Centro de Investigación Biomédica en Red de Enfermedades Hepáticas y Digestivas (CIBEREHD), Barcelona, Spain

6 Facultad de Medicina, Universidad International de Cataluña, Barcelona, Spain

*Address all correspondence to: cperalta@clinic.ub.es

References

[1] Baumann AJ, Wheeler DS, James M, Turner R, Siegel A, Navarro VJ. Benefit of early palliative care intervention in end-stage liver disease patients awaiting liver transplantation. Journal of Pain and Symptom Management. 2015;**50**(6):882-886.e2. DOI: 10.1016/j.jpainsymman.2015.07.014

[2] Knaak J, McVey M, Bazerbachi F, Goldaracena N, Spetzler V, Selzner N, et al. Liver transplantation in patients with end-stage liver disease requiring intensive care unit admission and intubation. Liver Transplantation. 2015;**21**(6):761-767. DOI: 10.1002/lt.24115

[3] Jimenez-Castro M, Elias-Miró M, Peralta C. Expanding the donor pool in liver transplantation: Influence of ischemia-reperfusion. In: Saidi RF, editor. Organ Donation and Organ Donors: Issues. New York: NOVA Science Publishers, Inc; 2013. p. 41-82

[4] Busuttil RW, Tanaka K. The utility of marginal donors in liver transplantation. Liver Transplantation. 2003;**9**(7): 651-663. DOI: 10.1053/jlts.2003.50105

[5] Gallegos-Orozco JF, Vargas HE, Rakela J. Virologically compromised donor grafts in liver transplantation. Journal of Hepatology. 2004;**41**(4): 512-521. DOI: 10.1016/j.jhep.2004.08.003

[6] Bacchella T, Galvão FHF, Almeida JLJ, Figueira ER, Moraes A, Machado MCC. Marginal grafts increase early mortality in liver transplantation. São Paulo Medical Journal. 2008;**126**(3):161-165. DOI: 10.1590/S1516-31802008000300005

[7] Lavanchy D. Hepatitis B virus epidemiology, disease burden, treatment, and current and emerging prevention and control measures. Journal of Viral Hepatitis. 2004;**11**(2):97-107. DOI: 10.1046/j.1365-2893.2003.00487.x

[8] Prieto M, Gómez MD, Berenguer M, Córdoba J, Rayón JM, Pastor M, et al. De novo hepatitis B after liver transplantation from hepatitis B core antibody-positive donors in an area with high prevalence of anti-HBc positivity in the donor population. Liver Transplantation. 2001;**7**(1):51-58. DOI: 10.1053/jlts.2001.20786

[9] Nickkholgh A, Weitz J, Encke J, Sauer P, Mehrabi A, Büchler MW, et al. Utilization of extended donor criteria in liver transplantation: A comprehensive review of the literature. Nephrology Dialysis Transplantation. 2007;**22**(s8):viii29-viii36. DOI: 10.1093/ndt/gfm654

[10] Dickson RC, Everhart JE, Lake JR, Wei Y, Seaberg EC, Wiesner RH, et al. Transmission of hepatitis B by transplantation of livers from donors positive for antibody to hepatitis B core antigen. The National Institute of Diabetes and Digestive and Kidney Diseases Liver Transplantation Database. Gastroenterology. 1997;**113**(5):1668-1674. DOI: 10.1053/gast.1997.v113.pm9352871

[11] Roth D, Fernandez JA, Babischkin S, De Mattos A, Buck BE, Quan S, et al. Detection of hepatitis C virus infection among cadaver organ donors: Evidence for low transmission of disease. Annals of Internal Medicine. 1992;**117**(6):470-475

[12] Candinas D, Joller-Jemelka HI, Schlumpf R, Wicki A, Mutimer DJ, Keusch G, et al. Hepatitis C RNA prevalence in a Western European organ donor pool and virus transmission by organ transplantation. Journal of Medical Microbiology. 1994;**41**(4):220-223. DOI: 10.1099/00222615-41-4-220

[13] Trotter JF. Expanding the donor pool for liver transplantation.

Current Gastroenterology Reports. 2000;**2**(1):46-54

[14] López-Navidad A, Caballero F. Extended criteria for organ acceptance. Strategies for achieving organ safety and for increasing organ pool. Clinical Transplantation. 2003;**17**(4):308-324

[15] Jiménez-Castro MB, Gracia-Sancho J, Peralta C. Brain death and marginal grafts in liver transplantation. Cell Death & Disease. 2015;**6**:e1777. DOI: 10.1038/cddis.2015.147

[16] Roque-Afonso AM, Feray C, Samuel D, Simoneau D, Roche B, Emile JF, et al. Antibodies to hepatitis B surface antigen prevent viral reactivation in recipients of liver graftsfrom anti-HBC positive donors. Gut. 2002;**50**(1):95-99

[17] Yu L, Koepsell T, Manhart L, Ioannou G. Survival after orthotopic liver transplantation: The impact of antibody against hepatitis B core antigen in the donor. Liver Transplantation. 2009;**15**(10):1343-1350. DOI: 10.1002/lt.21788

[18] Velidedeoglu E, Desai NM, Campos L, Olthoff KM, Shaked A, Nunes F, et al. The outcome of liver grafts procured from hepatitis C-positive donors. Transplantation. 2002;**73**(4):582-587

[19] Mukherjee S, Sorrell MF. Controversies in liver transplantation for hepatitis C. Gastroenterology. 2008;**134**(6):1777-1788. DOI: 10.1053/j.gastro.2008.02.035

[20] Castells L, Vargas V, Rodríguez-Frías F, Allende H, Jardí R, Margarit C, et al. Transmission of hepatitis B virus by transplantation of livers from donors positive for antibody to hepatitis B core antigen. Transplantation Proceedings. 1999;**31**(6):2464-5246

[21] Dodson SF, Issa S, Araya V, Gayowski T, Pinna A, Eghtesad B, et al. Infectivity of hepatic allografts with antibodies to hepatitis B virus. Transplantation. 1997;**64**(11):1582-1584

[22] Dodson SF, Bonham CA, Geller DA, Cacciarelli TV, Rakela J, Fung JJ. Prevention of de novo hepatitis B infection in recipients of hepatic allografts from anti-HBc positive donors. Transplantation. 1999;**68**(7):1058-1061

[23] Douglas DD, Rakela J, Wright TL, Krom RA, Wiesner RH. The clinical course of transplantation-associated de novo hepatitis B infection in the liver transplant recipient. Liver Transplantation and Surgery. 1997;**3**(2):105-111

[24] Lowell JA, Howard TK, White HM, Shenoy S, Huettner PC, Brennan DC, et al. Serological evidence of past hepatitis B infection in liver donor and hepatitis B infection in liver allograft. Lancet. 1995;**345**(8957):1084-1085

[25] Roche B, Samuel D, Gigou M, Feray C, Virot V, Schmets L, et al. De novo and apparent de novo hepatitis B virus infection after liver transplantation. Journal of Hepatology. 1997;**26**(3):517-526

[26] Smith H, Gibbs P. Hepatitis B, the hidden danger in cadaveric organ donors. Transplantation. 2000;**69**(3):458-459

[27] Uemoto S, Inomata Y, Sannomiya A, Koshiba T, Kurokawa T, Takatsuki M, et al. Posttransplant hepatitis B infection in liver transplantation with hepatitis B core antibody-positive donors. Transplantation Proceedings. 1998;**30**(1):134-135

[28] Uemoto S, Sugiyama K, Marusawa H, Inomata Y, Asonuma K, Egawa H, et al. Transmission of hepatitis B virus from hepatitis B core antibody-positive donors in living related liver transplants. Transplantation. 1998;**65**(4):494-499

[29] Yu AS, Vierling JM, Colquhoun SD, Arnaout WS, Chan CK, Khanafshar E, et al. Transmission of hepatitis B infection from hepatitis B core antibody-positive liver allografts is prevented by lamivudine therapy. Liver Transplantation. 2001;**7**(6):513-517. DOI: 10.1053/jlts.2001.23911

[30] Van Thiel DH, De Maria N, Colantoni A, Friedlander L. Can hepatitis B core antibody positive livers be used safely for transplantation: Hepatitis B virus detection in the liver of individuals who are hepatitis B core antibody positive. Transplantation. 1999;**68**(4):519-522

[31] Tur-Kaspa R, Burk RD, Shaul Y, Shafritz DA. Hepatitis B virus DNA contains a glucocorticoid-responsive element. Proceedings of the National Academy of Sciences of the United States of America. 1986;**83**(6):1627-1631

[32] Bock CT, Tillmann HL, Maschek HJ, Manns MP, Trautwein C. A preS mutation isolated from a patient with chronic hepatitis B infection leads to virus retention and misassembly. Gastroenterology. 1997;**113**(6):1976-1982

[33] Trautwein C, Schrem H, Tillmann HL, Kubicka S, Walker D, Böker KH, et al. Hepatitis B virus mutations in the pre-S genome before and after liver transplantation. Hepatology. 1996;**24**(3):482-488

[34] Samuel D, Forns X, Berenguer M, Trautwein C, Burroughs A, Rizzetto M, et al. Report of the monothematic EASL conference on liver transplantation for viral hepatitis (Paris, France, January 12-14, 2006). Journal of Hepatology. 2006;**45**(1):127-143. DOI: 10.1016/j.jhep.2006.05.001

[35] Raimondo G, Navarra G, Mondello S, Costantino L, Colloredo G, Cucinotta E, et al. Occult hepatitis B virus in liver tissue of individuals without hepatic disease. Journal of Hepatology. 2008;**48**(5):743-746. DOI: 10.1016/j.jhep.2008.01.023

[36] Tandoi F, Romagnoli R, Martini S, Mazza E, Nada E, Cocchis D, et al. Outcomes of liver transplantation in simultaneously hepatitis B surface antigen and hepatitis C virus RNA positive recipients: The deleterious effect of donor hepatitis B core antibody positivity. Transplantation Proceedings. 2012;**44**(7):1960-1962. DOI: 10.1016/j.transproceed.2012.07.061

[37] Muñoz SJ. Use of hepatitis B core antibody-positive donors for liver transplantation. Liver Transplantation. 2002;**8**(10 Suppl 1):S82-S87. DOI: 10.1053/jlts.2002.35783

[38] Testa G, Goldstein RM, Netto G, Abbasoglu O, Brooks BK, Levy MF, et al. Long-term outcome of patients transplanted with livers from hepatitis C-positive donors. Transplantation. 1998;**65**(7):925-929

[39] Marroquin CE, Marino G, Kuo PC, Plotkin JS, Rustgi VK, Lu AD, et al. Transplantation of hepatitis C-positive livers in hepatitis C-positive patients is equivalent to transplanting hepatitis C-negative livers. Liver Transplantation. 2001;**7**(9):762-768

[40] Ghobrial RM, Steadman R, Gornbein J, Lassman C, Holt CD, Chen P, et al. A 10-year experience of liver transplantation for hepatitis C: Analysis of factors determining outcome in over 500 patients. Annals of Surgery. 2001;**234**(3):384-393

[41] Khapra AP, Agarwal K, Fiel MI, Kontorinis N, Hossain S, Emre S, et al. Impact of donor age on survival and fibrosis progression in patients with hepatitis C undergoingliver transplantation using HCV+ allografts. Liver Transplantation. 2006;**12**(10):1496-1503. DOI: 10.1002/lt.20849

[42] Wang W, Niu Y, Yue Y, Wang L, Liu Y, Chen H, et al. Selection of liver graft from HCV-positive donor and prognosis of liver transplant recipients. International Journal of Clinical and Experimental Pathology. 2016;**9**(10):10817-10823

[43] Brown RS. Hepatitis C and liver transplantation. Nature. 2005;**436**(7053):973-978. DOI: 10.1038/nature04083

[44] Gastaca M. Extended criteria donors in liver transplantation: Adapting donor quality and recipient. Transplantation Proceedings. 2009 Apr;**41**(3):975-979. DOI: 10.1016/j.transproceed.2009.02.016

[45] Jaeschke H. Mechanisms of reperfusion injury after warm ischemia of the liver. Journal of Hepato-Biliary-Pancreatic Surgery. 1998;**5**(4):402-408

[46] Teoh NC, Farrell GC. Hepatic ischemia reperfusion injury: Pathogenic mechanisms and basis for hepatoprotection. Journal of Gastroenterology and Hepatology. 2003;**18**(8):891-902

[47] Jaeschke H. Molecular mechanisms of hepatic ischemia-reperfusion injury and preconditioning. American Journal of Physiology. Gastrointestinal and Liver Physiology. 2003;**284**(1):G15-G26

[48] Ploeg RJ, D'Alessandro AM, Knechtle SJ, Stegall MD, Pirsch JD, Hoffmann RM, et al. Risk factors for primary dysfunction after liver transplantation—A multivariate analysis. Transplantation. 1993;**55**(4):807-813

[49] Killackey MT, Gondolesi GE, Liu LU, Paramesh AS, Thung SN, Suriawinata A, et al. Effect of ischemia-reperfusion on the incidence of acute cellular rejection and timing of histologic hepatitis C virus recurrence after liver transplantation. Transplantation Proceedings. 2008;**40**(5):1504-1510. DOI: 10.1016/j.transproceed.2008.03.101

[50] Schemmer P, Mehrabi A, Kraus T, Sauer P, Gutt C, Uhl W, et al. New aspects on reperfusion injury to liver—Impact of organ harvest. Nephrology, Dialysis, Transplantation. 2004;**19** Suppl 4:iv26-iv35

[51] Kiuchi T, Oldhafer KJ, Schlitt HJ, Nashan B, Deiwick A, Wonigeit K, et al. Background and prognostic implications of perireperfusion tissue injuries in human livertransplants: A panel histochemical study. Transplantation. 1998;**66**(6):737-747

[52] Baron PW, Sindram D, Higdon D, Howell DN, Gottfried MR, Tuttle-Newhall JE, et al. Prolonged rewarming time during allograft implantation predisposes to recurrent hepatitis C infection after liver transplantation. Liver Transplantation. 2000;**6**(4):407-412

[53] Watt KD, Lyden ER, Gulizia JM, McCashland TM. Recurrent hepatitis C posttransplant: Early preservation injury may predict poor outcome. Liver Transplantation. 2006;**12**(1):134-139. DOI: 10.1002/lt.20583

[54] Velidedeoglu E, Mange KC, Frank A, Abt P, Desai NM, Markmann JW, et al. Factors differentially correlated with the outcome of liver transplantation in HCV+ and HCV− recipients. Transplantation. 2004;**77**(12):1834-1842

[55] Borghy-Scoazec G, Scoazec JY, Durand F, Bernuau J, Belghiti J, Feldmann G, et al. Apoptosis after ischemia-reperfusion in human liver allografts. Liver Transplantation and Surgery. 1997;**3**:407-415

[56] Ballardini G, De Raffele E, Groff P, Bioulac-Sage P, Grassi A, Ghetti S,

et al. Timing of reinfection and mechanisms of hepatocellular damage in transplanted hepatitis C virus-reinfected liver. Liver Transplantation. 2002;**8**(1):10-20. DOI: 10.1053/jlts.2002.30141

[57] Sung VM, Shimodaira S, Doughty AL, Picchio GR, Can H, Yen TS, et al. Establishment of B-cell lymphoma cell lines persistently infected with hepatitis C virus in vivo and in vitro: The apoptotic effects of virus infection. Journal of Virology. 2003;**77**(3):2134-2146

[58] Olthoff KM. Hepatic regeneration in living donor liver transplantation. Liver Transplantation. 2003;**9**(10 Suppl 2):S35-S41

[59] Molmenti EP, Klintmalm GBG. Hepatitis C recurrence after liver transplantation. Liver Transplantation. 2000;**6**(4):413-414. DOI: 10.1053/jlts.2000.8203

[60] Cameron AM, Ghobrial RM, Hiatt JR, Carmody IC, Gordon SA, Farmer DG, et al. Effect of nonviral factors on hepatitis C recurrence after liver transplantation. Annals of Surgery. 2006;**244**(4):563-571. DOI: 10.1097/01.sla.0000237648.90600.e9

[61] Crespo G, Mariño Z, Navasa M, Forns X. Viral hepatitis in liver transplantation. Gastroenterology. 2012;**142**(6):1373-1383.e1. DOI: 10.1053/j.gastro.2012.02.011

[62] Rosen HR, Hinrichs DJ, Gretch DR, Koziel MJ, Chou S, Houghton M, et al. Association of multispecific CD4(+) response to hepatitis C and severity of recurrence after livertransplantation. Gastroenterology. 1999;**117**(4):926-932

[63] Guo JT, Zhou H, Liu C, Aldrich C, Saputelli J, Whitaker T, et al. Apoptosis and regeneration of hepatocytes during recovery from transient hepadnavirus infections. Journal of Virology. 2000;**74**(3):1495-1505

[64] Rico MA, Quiroga JA, Subirá D, Garcia E, Castañón S, Sällberg M, et al. Features of the CD4+ T-cell response in liver and peripheral blood of hepatitis C virus-infected patients with persistently normal and abnormal alanine aminotransferase levels. Journal of Hepatology. 2002;**36**(3):408-416

[65] McCaughan GW, Zekry A. Mechanisms of HCV reinfection and allograft damage after liver transplantation. Journal of Hepatology. 2004;**40**(3):368-374

[66] Garcia-Retortillo M, Forns X, Feliu A, Moitinho E, Costa J, Navasa M, et al. Hepatitis C virus kinetics during and immediately after liver transplantation. Hepatology. 2002;**35**(3):680-687. DOI: 10.1053/jhep.2002.31773

[67] Guilera M, Forns X, Torras X, Enríquez J, Coll S, Solà R, et al. Pre-treatment with prednisolone does not improve the efficacy of subsequent alpha interferon therapy in chronic hepatitis C. Journal of Hepatology. 2000;**33**(1):135-141

[68] Tisone G, Angelico M, Palmieri G, Pisani F, Anselmo A, Baiocchi L, et al. A pilot study on the safety and effectiveness of immunosuppression without prednisone after liver transplantation. Transplantation. 1999;**67**(10):1308-1313

[69] McHutchison JG, Ponnudurai R, Bylund DL, Anguiano A, Pockros PJ, Mondala T, et al. Prednisone withdrawal followed by interferon alpha for treatment of chronic hepatitis C infection: Results of a randomized controlled trial. Journal of Clinical Gastroenterology. 2001;**32**(2):133-137

[70] Powers KA, Ribeiro RM, Patel K, Pianko S, Nyberg L, Pockros P, et al. Kinetics of hepatitis C virus reinfection after liver transplantation. Liver Transplantation. 2006;**12**(2):207-216. DOI: 10.1002/lt.20572

[71] Dahmen U, Li J, Dirsch O, Fiedler M, Lu M, Roggendorf M, et al. A new model of hepatitis B virus reinfection: Liver transplantation in the woodchuck1. Transplantation. 2002;**74**(3):373-380

[72] Dahmen U, Dirsch O, Li J, Fiedle M, Lu M, Rispeter K, et al. Adoptive transfer of immunity: A new strategy to interfere with severe hepatitis virus reinfection after woodchuck liver transplantation. Transplantation. 2004;**77**(7):965-972

[73] Uchiyama H, Yanaga K, Nishizaki T, Soejima Y, Yoshizumi T, Sugimachi K. Effects of deletion variant of hepatocyte growth factor on reduced-size liver transplantation in ratsTransplantation. 1999;**68**(1):39-44

[74] Cornide-Petronio ME, Casillas-Ramírez A, Jiménez-Castro MB, Peralta C. Experimental brain death models in liver transplantation. In: Tsoulfas G, editor. Organ Donation and Transplantation. London: IntechOpen; 2018. pp. 136-151

[75] Gracia-Sancho J, Casillas-Ramírez A, Peralta C. Molecular pathways in protecting the liver from ischaemia/reperfusion injury: A 2015 update. Clinical Science (London, England). 2015;**129**(4):345-362. DOI: 10.1042/CS20150223

[76] Chen YS, Wang CC, de Villa VH, Wang SH, Cheng YF, Huang TL, et al. Prevention of de novo hepatitis B virus infection in living donor liver transplantation using hepatitis B core antibody positive donors. Clinical Transplantation. 2002;**16**(6):405-409

[77] Manzarbeitia C, Reich DJ, Ortiz JA, Rothstein KD, Araya VR, Munoz SJ. Safe use of livers from donors with positive hepatitis B core antibody. Liver Transplantation. 2002;**8**(6):556-561. DOI: 10.1053/jlts.2002.33451

[78] Nery JR, Nery-Avila C, Reddy KR, Cirocco R, Weppler D, Levi DM, et al. Use of liver grafts from donors positive for antihepatitis B-core antibody (anti-HBc) in the era of prophylaxis with hepatitis-B immunoglobulin and lamivudine. Transplantation. 2003;**75**(8):1179-1186

[79] Prakoso E, Strasser SI, Koorey DJ, Verran D, McCaughan GW. Long-term lamivudine monotherapy prevents development of hepatitis B virus infection in hepatitis B surface-antigen negative liver transplant recipients from hepatitis B core-antibody-positive donors. Clinical Transplantation. 2006;**20**(3):369-373. DOI: 10.1111/j.1399-0012.2006.00495.x

[80] Fábrega E, García-Suarez C, Guerra A, Orive A, Casafont F, Crespo J, et al. Liver transplantation with allografts from hepatitis B core antibody-positive donors: A new approach. Liver Transplantation. 2003;**9**(9):916-920. DOI: 10.1053/jlts.2003.50190

[81] Kwon CHD, Suh KS, Yi NJ, Chang SH, Cho YB, Cho JY, et al. Long-term protection against hepatitis B in pediatric liver recipients can be achieved effectively with vaccination after transplantation. Pediatric Transplantation. 2006;**10**(4):479-486. DOI: 10.1111/j.1399-3046.2006.00540.x

[82] Umeda M, Marusawa H, Ueda M, Takada Y, Egawa H, Uemoto S, et al. Beneficial effects of short-term lamivudine treatment for de novo hepatitis B virus reactivation after liver transplantation. American Journal of Transplantation. 2006;**6**(11):2680-2685. DOI: 10.1111/j.1600-6143.2006.01542.x

[83] Suehiro T, Shimada M, Kishikawa K, Shimura T, Soejima Y, Yoshizumi T, et al. Prevention of hepatitis B virus infection from hepatitis B core antibody-positive donor graft using hepatitis B immune globulin and lamivudine in living donor liver transplantation. Liver International. 2005;**25**(6):1169-1174. DOI: 10.1111/j.1478-3231.2005.01165.x

[84] Hwang S, Lee SG, Park KM, Kim KH, Ahn CS, Oh HB, et al. Five-year follow-up of a hepatitis B virus-positive recipient of hepatitis B surface antigen-positive living donor liver graft. Liver Transplantation. 2006;**12**(6):993-997. DOI: 10.1002/lt.20799

[85] Chhatwal J, Samur S, Bethea ED, Ayer T, Kanwal F, Hur C, et al. Transplanting hepatitis C virus-positive livers into hepatitis C virus-negative patients with preemptive antiviral treatment: A modeling study. Hepatology. 2018;**67**(6):2085-2095. DOI: 10.1002/hep.29723

[86] Campos-Varela I, Agudelo EZ, Sarkar M, Roberts JP, Terrault NA. Use of a hepatitis C virus (HCV) RNA-positive donor in a treated HCV RNA-negative liver transplant recipient. Transplant Infectious Disease. 2018;**20**(1):1-8. DOI: 10.1111/tid.12809

[87] Saberi B, Hamilton JP, Durand CM, Li Z, Philosophe B, Cameron AM, et al. Utilization of hepatitis C virus RNA-positive donor liver for transplant to hepatitis C virus RNA-negative recipient. Liver Transplantation. 2018;**24**(1):140-143. DOI: 10.1002/lt.24838